Sous Vide Cookbook

Modern Recipes Made Easy

Jenny Glover

Table of Contents

Introduction

It is not only the French name that makes it fancy. Sous vide cooking in machines that are specially designed for that purpose results in elegant, restaurant-like dishes that leave everyone breathless. But don't get overwhelmed by the high degree of quality. You don't have to be an experienced chef to sous vide cook. Beginners can also master this cooking method, and this book will show you how.

No matter which sous vide machine you've bought, the cooking method is pretty much the same. And while the dishes you will be making with your sous vide machine will be of high-quality, know that there is nothing too special about the cooking process. In fact, it is straightforward and easy. Dive deeply into this book and find out for yourself.

Providing you with 150 different delicacies and yummy dishes, this book will enrich your recipe folder with delightful breakfast dishes, appetizers and snacks, poultry dishes, beef delicacies, egg recipes, stocks and sauces, and desserts.

And the best part? The instructions are so simple, you will become a sous vide master in no time.

Sound like a good deal? Try these mouth-watering recipes and see that sous vide is the master of taste.

Bon Appetit!

Sous Vide Tools

The great thing about cooking sous vide with the Joule is that you don't need a lot of complicated cooking equipment. The Joule is the most versatile sous vide unit on the market partly because it allows you to cook in almost any container. Typically, you would use a Plexiglas Cambro vessel to cook sous vide, but the Joule allows you to cook in a large bowl, the kitchen sink, or anything that holds enough water to fully submerge the food you would like to cook.

Other than maintaining a constant temperature, the other important feature of sous vide cooking is the "vide" or vacuum. In order for your food to cook evenly, it needs to have even contact with the water bath. For this reason, you will need to use a method for sealing the food in a plastic bag. Simple food sealing devices like the FoodSaver® or Seal-a-Meal® make the process fast, easy, and reliable. But if you don't feel like purchasing another piece of equipment, you can achieve a good seal using the water displacement method. Simply place your food in a zipper locked bag and seal all but a small corner of the zipper lock. Then, slowly submerge the bag in the water bath (make sure the water isn't too hot when you do this). As you submerge the bag, the air will be forced out through the unsealed corner of the bag. When only this corner is above the surface of the water, pinch the zipper lock shut, and all of the air will be removed.

NOTE: When choosing zipper lock bags, make sure to check the packaging to make sure the bags are BPA free. Because the dangers of BPA are now well known, most bags are already certified BPA free and are safe to use for sous vide cooking.

Sous Vide Cooking

Sous vide, which means *under vacuum* in French, is the process of vacuuming the food, usually in a bag, and cooking in water at a very precise temperature. This may seem fancy, but other than the fancy dishes, there is nothing complex about the cooking method. The process is super simple, and it involves only three cooking steps:

1. Attach the sous vide machine to a pot of water, and set the exact cooking temperature. If using an all-in-one sous vide machine that has an attached container, you only need to fill it up with water and set the cooking temperature.

2. Place the food in a sealable bag, get rid of the excess air, and seal it.

3. Immerse the bag in the preheated water, and cook for as long as you need to get the best results.

If you want to add a crispy exterior layer, you can finish your food by searing or grilling it.

Why Sous Vide?

Sous vide is probably the most precise cooking method, thanks to the circulation of the temperature. There is no other cooking machine on the market that can offer similar results. Because it has a cooking technique that can be controlled down to a single degree, this cooking method offers the tenderest and most flavorful dishes you will ever taste.

Let's take steak for example. If you are like me, you like your steak cooked to perfection, which can never be done with pan-searing. Think about it; no matter how much you try, you will always end up with edges that are much more overcooked than the center. And if you don't want to overcook the edges, you end up with a very pink center – which I personally hate. Now, how can sous vide help? With this cooking method, there is absolutely no gradient in color. You can choose to set your temperature to 135 degrees F and cook the steak for 2 hours. The end result is a perfectly-cooked steak that it is exactly 135 F. If you want it to be crispier, simply sear it for a minute on the stove, and problem solved.

The Benefits

Consistency – Thanks to the extremely precise cooking temperature, you can expect results that are super consistent.

Incredibly tasty – Here, the food cooks in its own juices. You don't have to marinate your meat for hours prior to cooking. Why? Because you will be cooking it in marinade. Simply dump everything in a bag, seal it, immerse in the water, and let the sous vide machine do its thing.

Volume increase – Don't you just hate it when your piece of meat shrinks by half during the cooking process? With sous vide cooking, the food doesn't lose its volume. Still in doubt? Take two equal cuts of steak. Cook one traditionally and the other one sealed in a bag with your sous vide machine. The traditionally-cooked steak will lose a minimum of 40 percent of its volume, while the sous vide steak will keep its original shape and size.

Flexibility – There is absolutely no stirring or whisking involved. You simply immerse the bag with food, set the cooking temperature, tie it, and forget about it. You don't need to worry about the cooking process at all. You can let it cook overnight and enjoy tasty breakfast in the morning.

Money saving – You don't have to purchase the most expensive cut of meat to wow your guests. Sous vide cooking can cook every meat cut to perfection, providing you with a high-quality dish ready to be served.

What Do You Need?

In order for you to prevent evaporation and ensure that the energy transfer from the water to the food will be consistent and efficient, your food must be sealed well. However, you don't have to go all crazy and buy the most expensive vacuum sealer there is. In fact, you don't even need a vacuum sealer.

Here is the most beneficial packaging for sous vide cooking:

Ziploc Bags

Ziploc bags are resealable, versatile, and very useful for this cooking technique. And the best part? You can easily seal it with the water immersion method. Simply fill your bag with the food, liquids, and all the seasoning, and immerse it in the preheated water, but not all the way. Notice how the excess air of the immersed part has gone. Once you have vacuumed your food, you can simply seal the bag, and that's it.

When using zipper locked bags, make sure they are of high quality and are BPA-free for your own safety.

Silicone Bags

If you are not a fan of plastic, you can choose resealable silicone bags instead. The cooking and sealing method here is the same.

Vacuum Sealing Bags

Like I said, you don't necessarily have to have a vacuum sealer to sous vide cook; however, keep in mind that these vacuum seal bags are the perfect choice for batch cooking. And if you have a large family, you may find them more than necessary.

Canning Jars

Who says you have to cook in bags only? Your sous vide machine can also cook food in jars and cook it to perfection. From beans and grains to cakes, muffins, and custards, there are a lot of food choices that can be cooked in jars.

Sous Vide Cooking Chart

Beef Steak, rare	129F	1 hr 30 min
Beef Steak, medium-rare	136F	1 hr 30 min
Beef Steak, well done	158F	1 hr 30 min
Beef Roast, rare	133F	7 hrs
Beef Roast, medium-rare	140F	6 hrs
Beef Roast, well done	158F	5 hrs
Beef Tough Cuts, rare	136F	24 hrs
Beef Tough Cuts, medium-rare	149F	16 hrs
Beef Tough Cuts, well done	185F	8 hrs
Lamb Tenderloin, Rib-eye	134F	4 hrs
T-bone, Cutlets	134F	4 hrs
Lamb Roast, Leg	134F	10 hrs
Lamb Flank Steak, Brisket	134F	12 hrs
Pork Chop, rare	136F	1 hr
Pork Chop, medium-rare	144F	1 hr
Pork Chop, well done	158F	1 hr
Pork Roast, rare	136F	3 hrs
Pork Roast, medium-rare	144F	3 hrs
Pork Roast, well done	158F	3 hrs
Pork Tough Cuts, rare	144F	16 hrs
Pork Tough Cuts, medium-rare	154F	12 hrs

Pork Tough Cuts, well done	180F	8 hrs
Pork Tenderloin	134F	1 hr 30 min
Pork Baby Back Ribs	165F	6 hrs
Pork Cutlets	134F	5 hrs
Scallops	140F	50 min
Shrimp	140F	35 min

Vegetables, root (carrots, potato, parsnips, beets, celery root, turnips) 183F 3 hrs

Vegetables, tender (asparagus, broccoli, cauliflower, fennel, onions, pumpkin, eggplant, green beans, corn) 183F 1 hr

Vegetables, greens (kale, spinach, collard greens, Swiss chard) 183F 5 min

Fruit, firm (apple, pear) 183F 45 min

Fruit, for puree 185F 30 min

Fruit, berries for topping to desserts (blueberries, blackberries, raspberries, strawberries) 154 30 min

Breakfast

Perfect Poached Eggs

Servings: 2 | Prep Time: 2 minutes | Cook Time: 45 minutes

Ingredients:
  2 large eggs

Instructions:

1. Fill a water bath and set your Joule to 145F/62C.
2. Submerge the eggs and cook for 45 minutes. When eggs are nearly cooked, heat a small pot of water to boiling.
3. Remove the eggs from the water bath, and gently remove the shells. Place the eggs in the boiling water for 10 seconds and carefully remove them. For a slightly firmer yolk, boil an additional 15 seconds.

Nutritional Info: Calories: 72, Sodium: 70 mg, Dietary Fiber: 0 g, Fat: 5 g, Carbs: 7.4 g, Protein: 6.3 g.

Ham and Egg Scramble

Servings: 4 | Prep time: 10 minutes | Cook time: 40 minutes

Ingredients:

8 large eggs
1/4-pound Black Forest ham
1/2 cup sharp cheddar cheese, grated
2 tablespoons butter, melted
1/2 teaspoon salt
1/2 cup whole milk

Instructions:

1. Fill a water bath and set your Joule to 170F/76C.
2. In a medium bowl, scramble the eggs and add the ham, cheese, butter, salt, and milk. Mix well and pour into a zipper lock bag. Remove all air from the bag and place in the water bath for 20 minutes.
3. Remove the bag from the water bath and, using your hands, mix the contents. Then place back in the water bath for an additional 20 minutes. Remove the bag from the water bath and serve immediately.

Nutritional Info: Calories: 315, Sodium: 941 mg, Dietary Fiber: 0.4 g, Fat: 23.8 g, Carbs: 3.4 g, Protein: 21.9 g.

Sous Vide French Toast

Servings: 4 | Prep time: 10 minutes | Cook time: 60
minutes

Ingredients:

8 large eggs
3/4 cups milk
1 teaspoon vanilla extract
1/2 teaspoon salt
4 thick slices of bread
2 tablespoons butter

Instructions:

1. Fill a water bath and set your Joule to 147F/67C.
2. In a large bowl, combine the eggs, milk, vanilla, and salt, and mix well. Soak the bread in the egg mixture and place in a zipper lock bag. Remove all the air from the bag and submerge in the water bath for 60 minutes.
3. When you're almost finished cooking, heat a skillet with the butter over medium heat. Remove the bread from the water bath and place in the skillet until lightly browned on each side. Serve immediately with maple syrup or powdered sugar.

Nutritional Info: Calories: 244, Sodium: 555 mg, Dietary Fiber: 0.2 g, Fat: 16.9 g, Carbs: 7.7 g, Protein: 14.8 g.

Classic Eggs Benedict

Servings: 4 | Prep time: 30 minutes | Cook time: 30 minutes

Ingredients:
4 eggs, poached
4 slices Black Forest or tavern ham
4 English muffins, toasted
For the sauce:
1 cup white wine
3 tablespoons champagne or white wine vinegar
1 teaspoon fresh thyme
6 egg yolks
1 cup unsalted butter, melted
1 tablespoon lemon juice

Instructions:

1. Fill a water bath and set your Joule to 145F/62C.
2. In a medium saucepan heat the wine, vinegar, and thyme until boiling and simmer for 10 minutes. Remove from heat and pour into a blender with the egg yolks and puree until smooth.
3. Pour the mixture into a large zipper lock bag and submerge in the water bath for 30 minutes.
4. While the Hollandaise sauce cooks, poach the eggs and toast the muffins. Remove the Hollandaise sauce from the water bath and stir. You can also keep the sauce in the water bath for up to 2 hours if you're not ready to serve right away.
5. To assemble, Place the muffins on plates, top with ham, a poached egg, and cover with Hollandaise sauce. Garnish with chopped chives and serve immediately.

Nutritional Info: Calories: 752, Sodium: 740 mg, Dietary Fiber: 2.1 g, Fat: 58.7 g, Carbs: 28.9 g, Protein: 15.7 g.

Red Pepper Frittata

Servings: 3 | Prep time: 30 minutes | Cook time: 60 minutes

Ingredients:

6 large eggs
1 red bell pepper, diced
1 teaspoon salt
1 tablespoon butter
3 tablespoons yellow onion, finely chopped
1/4 cup milk
1/2 teaspoon red pepper flakes

Instructions:

1. Fill a water bath and set your Joule to 176F/80C.
2. In a medium skillet over medium heat, melt the butter and add the bell pepper, onion, and pepper flakes. Cook until the onions and peppers are tender. Remove from heat.
3. In a large bowl, scramble the eggs and add the salt, onion and pepper mixture, and milk. Stir well and pour into 3 mason jars. Secure the lids and submerge in the water bath for 60 minutes.
4. Remove the jars from the water bath and allow to cool slightly before servings.

Nutritional Info: Calories: 205, Sodium: 953 mg, Dietary Fiber: 0.8 g, Fat: 14.4 g, Carbs: 5.9 g, Protein: 13.8 g.

Canadian Bacon

Servings: 8 | Prep time: 5 minutes | Cook time: 6 to 12 hours

Ingredients:
>   *8 thick slices tavern ham*
>   *1 teaspoon vegetable oil*

Instructions:

1. Fill a water bath and set your Joule to 145F/62C.
2. Place the ham slices side by side in a large zipper lock bag and remove all of the air from the bag.
3. Submerge the bag in the water bath for at least 6 and up to 12 hours.
4. Heat a large skillet with the oil and remove the ham from the water bath. Place each slice of ham onto the skillet and cook, pressing down on the ham with a spatula until lightly browned.
5. Serve immediately.

Nutritional Info: Calories: 24, Sodium: 93 mg, Dietary Fiber: 0 g, Fat: 0.6 g, Carbs: 0.3 g, Protein: 3 g.

Scotch Eggs

Prep time: 2 hours
Cooking time: 54 minutes
Servings: 4

Ingredients:

4 eggs
1 cup breadcrumbs
7 oz. ground beef
1 teaspoon salt
1 teaspoon ground black pepper
1 teaspoon paprika
½ cup flour
1 teaspoon dried cilantro
1 cup olive oil

Directions:

1. Put the eggs in the plastic bag.
2. Set the Sous Vide machine at 145 C and preheat the water.
3. Then put the plastic bag with the eggs in the preheated water and cook it for 45 minutes.
4. Meanwhile, combine the ground beef with the salt, ground black pepper, paprika, and dried dill.
5. Mix the ground beef carefully with the help of the fingertips.
6. When the time is over and eggs are cooked – remove them from the Sous Vide saucepan and chill little.
7. After this, put the eggs in the freezer and freeze them for at least 1 hour.
8. Then peel the eggs.
9. Dip the peeled eggs in the flour.
10. Then coat them with the ground meat mixture.
11. Then sprinkle the coated eggs with the breadcrumbs.
12. Leave the prepared eggs for 1 hour.

13. Meanwhile, pour the olive oil into the saucepan and preheat it until the oil is boiled.
14. After 1 hour, put the coated eggs in the boiling olive oil and cook those for 5-7 minutes or till the scotch eggs are cooked.
15. Dry the scotch eggs with the help of the paper towel gently.
16. Enjoy!

Nutrition: calories 858, fat 79.1, fiber 1, carbs 19, protein 19

Starbucks Egg Bites

Prep time: 20 minutes
Cooking time: 1 hour
Servings: 4

Ingredients:

¼ cup cottage cheese
4 egg whites
1 tablespoon chives
1 sweet red pepper
1 teaspoon olive oil
3 tablespoon spinach
1 teaspoon cornstarch
¼ teaspoon hot sauce
1 teaspoon butter
1/3 teaspoon ground black pepper
¼ teaspoon salt

Directions:

1. Whisk the eggs whites until they are homogenous.
2. Then add the cottage cheese and continue to whisk it for 30 seconds more.
3. After this, discard the seeds from the sweet red pepper and chop it.
4. Add the chopped sweet pepper in the whisked egg white mixture.
5. Add the cornstarch and hot sauce.
6. After this, sprinkle the egg white mixture with the salt and ground black pepper.
7. Chop the spinach and chives and add the ingredients in the egg white mixture.
8. Whisk the mixture gently again and add butter.
9. Spray the small glass jars with the olive oil.
10. Then fill the 1/3 of every glass jar with the mixed egg white mixture. Close the lids.

11. Set the Sous Vide machine in the saucepan and add water there.
12. Set the Sous Vide machine at 172 F.
13. When the water is preheated, put the closed glass jars in the saucepan and cook the egg bites for 1 hour.
14. Meanwhile, preheat the oven to 360 F.
15. Cover the tray with the parchment.
16. When the egg bites are cooked – remove them from the glass jars gently and transfer to the prepared tray.
17. Put the tray in the preheated oven and broil the dish for 4-7 minutes.
18. After this, let the prepared egg bites chill gently.
19. Serve it!

Nutrition: calories 58, fat 2.8, fiber 0, carbs 2.86, protein 5

Breakfast Bacon

Prep time: 15 minutes
Cooking time: 9 hours
Servings: 4

Ingredients:

1-pound bacon
1 teaspoon salt
½ teaspoon dried oregano
½ teaspoon turmeric
½ teaspoon ground paprika
½ teaspoon ground black pepper
½ teaspoon chili pepper

Directions:

1. Slice the bacon.
2. Combine the salt, dried oregano, turmeric, ground paprika, ground black pepper, and chili pepper together in the shallow bowl.
3. Mix it gently with the help of the fork.
4. Then rub every bacon slice with the spice mixture carefully.
5. Put the sliced bacon in the plastic bag and vacuum it.
6. Set the Sous Vide machine at 145 F.
7. When the water is preheated to the adjusted temperature – put the vacuumed sliced bacon there.
8. Cook the bacon for 9 hours.
9. After this, preheat the skillet well.
10. Put the Sous Vide bacon in the preheated skillet and roast it for 20 seconds from each side.
11. Serve the bacon hot.

Nutrition: calories 359, fat 33.6, fiber 3, carbs 8.73, protein 12

Tomato Egg Bites

Prep time: 10 minutes
Cooking time: 1 hour
Servings: 5

Ingredients:

5 eggs
2 tomatoes
1 teaspoon salt
¼ cup cream
½ teaspoon canola oil
¼ teaspoon ground white pepper
½ teaspoon cilantro
2 tablespoon fresh parsley
¼ teaspoon ground paprika

Directions:

1. Beat the eggs in the big bowl and whisk them well.
2. Then wash the tomatoes and chop them.
3. Add the chopped tomatoes in the egg mixture.
4. Then add the cream, salt, ground white pepper, cilantro, and ground paprika.
5. Chop the fresh cilantro and add it to the egg mixture.
6. Stir the egg mixture gently.
7. Take the glass jars and sprinkle them with the canola oil.
8. Pour the egg mixture into the glass jars to fill the ½ of every vessel.
9. Close every glass jar with the lid.
10. Then set the Sous Vide machine at 172 F.
11. Put the glass jars in the saucepan with the Sous Vide equipment and cook the egg bites for 1 hour.
12. When the time is over and the egg bites are cooked – remove them from the glass jars and serve.
13. Enjoy!

Nutrition: calories 168, fat 12.6, fiber 1, carbs 3.74, protein 10

Egg Cups with Bacon

Prep time: 15 minutes
Cooking time: 55 minutes
Servings: 5

Ingredients:

5 eggs
4 oz. bacon, cooked
1 tablespoon cream cheese
½ teaspoon salt
½ teaspoon ground white pepper
¼ teaspoon chili flakes
1 teaspoon olive oil
1 tablespoon chives

Directions:

1. Take the ramekins and spray them with the olive oil inside.
2. After this, crack the eggs in the prepared ramekins.
3. Chop the chives.
4. Combine the salt, cream cheese, ground white pepper, and chili flakes in the separated bowl.
5. Add the chopped chives and mix the mixture up.
6. After this, add the small amount of the cream cheese mixture in the ramekins with the cracked eggs.
7. Preheat the Sous Vide saucepan till 145 F.
8. Then cover the ramekins with the plastic paper.
9. Put the prepared ramekins in the saucepan and cook the dish for 55 minutes.
10. When the eggs are cooked but still soft – the dish is cooked.
11. Serve the breakfast immediately.
12. Enjoy!

Nutrition: calories 219, fat 18.1, fiber 1, carbs 3.07, protein 12

Delightful Oatmeal

Prep time: 7 minutes
Cooking time: 9 hours
Servings: 3

Ingredients:

2 tablespoon brown sugar
1 teaspoon vanilla extract
1 cup oatmeal
1 cup milk
¼ teaspoon salt
¼ teaspoon ground ginger
¼ teaspoon ground cardamom
2 teaspoon honey

Directions:

1. Put the oatmeal, salt, brown sugar, ground ginger, and the ground cardamom in the plastic Sous Vide bag.
2. Shake it gently and add the vanilla extract, milk, and honey.
3. Seal the bag.
4. Set the Sous Vide to 180 F and put the sealed bag with the oatmeal mixture there.
5. Cook the oatmeal for 9 hours or overnight.
6. When the oatmeal is cooked – remove it from the sealed bag and transfer to the serving bowls.
7. Mix it gently with the help of the spoon and enjoy!

Nutrition: calories 163, fat 3.5, fiber 2, carbs 29.03, protein 4

Breakfast Mini Cheesecakes

Prep time: 12 minutes
Cooking time: 91 minute
Servings: 5

Ingredients:

½ cup cream cheese
3 eggs
4 tablespoon white sugar
½ teaspoon vanilla extract
5 tablespoon cottage cheese
1 teaspoon orange zest

Directions:

1. Beat the eggs in the mixer bowl and mix them carefully.
2. Then add the white sugar, cream cheese, vanilla extract, cottage, and orange zest.
3. Mix the mixture very carefully until you get the smooth and soft texture.
4. After this, take the mason jars and fill the ½ part of every jar.
5. Set the Sous Vide to 176 F and put the mason jars there.
6. Cook the mini cheesecakes for 91 minute.
7. When the cheesecakes are cooked – chill them little and put the fridge to make them chill totally.
8. Serve the dish!

Nutrition: calories 166, fat 13.3, fiber 0, carbs 2.38, protein 9

Egg Yolk Croquettes

Prep time: 20 minutes
Cooking time: 50 minutes
Servings: 5

Ingredients:

5 egg yolks
2 eggs
1 cup panko bread crumbs
5 tablespoon flour
3 tablespoon olive oil
½ teaspoon salt
¼ teaspoon dried oregano
¼ teaspoon ground paprika

Directions:

1. Set the Sous Vide machine to 148 F.
2. Then put the egg yolks in the Sous Vide machine without any bag and cook them for 45 minutes.
3. Turn the eggs into another side with the help of the silicone spatula after 26 minutes of cooking.
4. Meanwhile, beat the egg in the bowl and whisk it carefully.
5. Add the flour, salt, and dried oregano.
6. Whisk the mixture well.
7. When the egg yolks are cooked – let them chill little.
   a. After this, dip the egg yolks in the egg-flour mixture.
8. Then coat the egg yolks in the panko bread crumbs.
9. Pour the olive oil in the pan and preheat it.
10. Then put the egg yolk croquettes in the preheated olive oil and roast them for 5-7 minutes. Flip them into other sides during the cooking.
11. Then put the prepared egg yolk croquettes on the serving plate and sprinkle with the ground paprika.
12. Serve it!

Nutrition: calories 226, fat 16.8, fiber 1, carbs 10.55, protein 8

Breakfast Coffee Butter Slices

Prep time: 10 minutes
Cooking time: 3 hours
Servings: 4

Ingredients:

> *6 tablespoon coffee*
> *12 tablespoon butter*
> *6 oz. white bread*
> *1 teaspoon brown sugar*
> *½ teaspoon ground cinnamon*

Directions:

1. Put the coffee in the plastic bag.
2. Add butter and brown sugar.
3. Add the ground cinnamon and seal the plastic bag.
4. Set the Sous Vide to 195 F.
5. When the water is preheated – put the sealed bag there and cook the coffee butter for 3 hours.
6. After this, remove the coffee butter from the Sous Vide and chill it for 4 minutes.
7. Then strain the coffee butter. Do it fast till the butter is still liquid.
   a. Then place the coffee butter in the butter mold and freeze it in the freezer.
8. When the coffee butter is solid – it is cooked.
9. Slice the white bread and spread it with the coffee butter.
10. Enjoy!

Nutrition: calories 412, fat 35.5, fiber 4, carbs 20.09, protein 5

Cocktails and Infusions

Cinnamon Quince Bourbon

(Prep + Cook Time: 2 hours and 20 minutes / Servings: 8)

Ingredients:

2 cups Bourbon

2 Quinces, peeled and sliced
1 Cinnamon Stick

Directions:

1. Preheat the Sous Vide to 150 degrees F.
2. Place all the ingredients in a Ziploc bag.
3. Seal and immerse in the water.
4. Cook for 2 hours.
5. Strain the bourbon through a cheesecloth.

Nutritional info per serving: Calories 143, Carbohydrates 3.5 g, Fat 0 g, Protein 0 g

Sous Vide Eggnog

(Prep + Cook Time: 1 hour and 30 minutes / Servings: 4)

Ingredients:

2 cups Milk

4 Eggs
¾ cup Sugar
½ cup Rum
1 cup Heavy Cream
½ tbsp Vanilla Extract
2 Cinnamon Sticks
Nutmeg, for serving

Directions:

1. Preheat the water to 140 degrees F.
2. Whisk all the ingredients in a jar or a Ziploc bag.
3. Seal and immerse in the water. Cook for 1 hour.
4. Strain through a coffee filter.
5. Serve sprinkled with ground nutmeg.

Nutritional info per serving: Calories 550, Carbohydrates 27 g, Fat 35 g, Protein 14 g

Gingery Gin and Tonic with Lemons
(Prep + Cook Time: 2 hours and 20 minutes / Servings: 4)

Ingredients:

1 cup Gin

1 cup Ice
1 ¼ cups Tonic Water
1 inch Ginger Piece, peeled
1 Lemon, cut into wedges

Directions:

4. Preheat the water to 125 degrees.
5. Place the gin, ginger, and half of the lemon wedges in a Ziploc bag.
6. Get rid of the excess air and seal.
7. Place in the water and cook for 2 hours.
8. Let cool completely.
9. Serve with ice and remaining lemon wedges.

Nutritional info per serving: Calories 630, Carbohydrates 30 g, Fat 0 g, Protein 0 g

Hot and Sweet Cinnamony Red Wine
(Prep + Cook Time: 4 hours and 10 minutes / Servings: 4)

Ingredients:

1 bottle of Red Wine

2 Cinnamon Sticks
1 Orange, cut in half
¼ cup Honey
1 cup Apple Cider
5 Whole Cloves
2 Star Anise

Directions:

1. Preheat your Sous Vide to 150 degrees F.
2. Place all the ingredients in a Ziploc bag.
3. Seal and immerse in the water.
4. Cook for 4 hours.
5. Serve hot.

Nutritional info per serving: Calories 270, Carbohydrates 33 g, Fat 0 g, Protein 0.5 g

Vanilla Coffee Liqueur

(Prep + Cook Time: 24 hours and 10 minutes / Servings: 8)

Ingredients:

1 ½ cups Vodka

1 cup Sugar
1 pound Coffee Beans
1 Vanilla Bean, split
½ cup Cacao Nibs

Directions:

1. Preheat the Sous Vide to 150 degrees F.
2. Combine everything in a Ziploc bag and get rid of the excess air.
3. Immerse the sealed bag in the preheated water.
4. Cook for 24 hours.

Nutritional info per serving: Calories 244, Carbohydrates 21 g, Fat 2.6 g, Protein 1 g

Side Dishes

Japanese Style Turnip

Prep time: 15 minutes
Cooking time: 32 minutes
Servings: 4

Ingredients

2 oz. water
3 oz. butter
1 tablespoon miso paste
1 tablespoon brown sugar
10 oz. turnip
1 tablespoon chives

Directions:

1. Melt the butter until it is soft but not melted.
2. Then combine the melted butter with the water and miso paste.
3. Add the brown sugar and mix the mixture up till the miso paste is dissolved.
4. Peel the turnip and slice it.
5. Put the sliced turnip in the plastic bag.
6. Add the miso paste mixture and close it.
7. Seal the plastic bag.
8. Preheat the Sous Vide water bath to 185 F and put the sealed plastic bag there.
9. Cook the turnip for 32 minutes.
10. Meanwhile, chop the chives.
11. Then preheat the skillet.
12. Remove the prepared turnip from the Sous Vide bath and transfer the content of the sealed bag in the preheated skillet.
13. Roast the turnip about 2 minutes on the medium heat.
14. Stir it frequently.
15. Transfer the prepared turnip in the serving plate and sprinkle with the chopped chives.

16. Serve it!

Nutrition: calories 186, fat 17.8, fiber 2, carbs 5, protein 3

Aromatic Fennel

Prep time: 15 minutes
Cooking time: 2 hours
Servings: 4

Ingredients

1-pound fennel bulb
1 teaspoon thyme
1 teaspoon ground coriander
1 teaspoon salt
1 tablespoon olive oil
1 tablespoon fresh parsley
4 oz. Cheddar cheese
1 teaspoon lemon juice

Directions:

1. Wash the fennel bulb carefully and cut it into 4 parts.
2. Put the fennel pieces in the Sous Vide plastic bag.
3. Add the thyme, ground coriander, salt, olive oil, and fresh parsley.
4. Close the plastic bag and shake it gently.
5. Prepare the Sous Vide water bath and preheat it to 177 F.
6. Seal the Sous Vide plastic bag and put it in the water bath.
7. Cook the fennel for 2 hours.
8. Meanwhile, shred Cheddar cheese.
9. When the fennel is cooked – remove it from the water bath and discard from the sealed bag.
10. Put the fennel pieces on the serving plates.
11. Sprinkle the side dish with the lemon juice and shredded Cheddar cheese.
12. Enjoy the side dish warm.

Nutrition: calories 116, fat 6.1, fiber 4, carbs 12, protein 5

Carrots

Prep time: 20 minutes
Cooking time: 1.5 hours
Servings: 4

Ingredients

1-pound medium carrots
3 tablespoon fresh cilantro
1 tablespoon fresh parsley
3 tablespoon water
1 tablespoon butter
1 teaspoon salt
1 tablespoon ground ginger
1 tablespoon maple syrup

Directions:

1. Wash the carrot carefully and peel it.
2. Then chop the fresh cilantro, fresh parsley, and combine the greens with the ground ginger and salt.
3. Mix the green carefully.
4. Put the peeled carrots in the plastic bag in a single layer.
5. Add the green mixture.
6. Then put the water, butter, and maple syrup.
7. Seal the plastic bag.
8. Preheat the Sous Vide water bath to 184 F and put the sealed plastic bag with the carrot there.
9. Cook the carrot for 1.5 hours.
10. Meanwhile, prepare the ice bath: combine the ice cubes and cold water in the big bowl.
11. When the time is over – put the sealed bag with the carrot in the ice bath and leave it for 3 minutes.
12. Then discard the carrot from the plastic bag and transfer the vegetables to the serving plates.
13. Serve the carrots!

Nutrition: calories 90, fat 3.2, fiber 3, carbs 15.24, protein 1

Sweet Carrot Puree

Prep time: 15 minutes
Cooking time: 2 hours
Servings: 8

Ingredients

2-pound carrot
½ cup milk
2 tablespoon butter
½ cup fresh dill
2 tablespoon sugar
1 teaspoon paprika
1 teaspoon salt
½ teaspoon fresh ginger
1 tablespoon heavy cream
1 apple

Directions:

1. Peel the carrot and chop it.
2. Put the chopped carrot in the plastic bag.
3. Add the butter, fresh dill, sugar, paprika, salt, fresh ginger, heavy cream, and milk.
4. Peel the apple and discard the seeds.
5. Add the prepared apple in the plastic bag too.
6. After this, close the plastic bag and seal it.
7. Set Sous Vide water bath to 190 F and put the sealed bag with the carrot there.
8. Cook the dish for 2 hours.
9. When the dish is cooked – remove it from the water bath.
10. Then transfer the content of the plastic bag in the blender and blend it until you get the soft carrot puree.
11. Use the puff pastry bag and nozzle to serve it on the serving plates.
12. Enjoy!

Nutrition: calories 102, fat 4.4, fiber 4, carbs 15, protein 2

Garlic Artichokes

Prep time: 25 minutes
Cooking time: 2 hours
Servings: 5

Ingredients

3 medium artichokes
1 cup garlic, peeled
3 lemons
3 tablespoon garlic sauce
1 tablespoon green onion
1 tablespoon mustard
4 tablespoon olive oil

Directions:

1. Wash the artichokes and prepare them for cooking.
2. Then put the artichokes in the saucepan.
3. Cut the lemons into the halves and squeeze the lemon juice over the prepared artichokes.
4. Mince the garlic and add it to the saucepan with the artichokes.
5. After this, add the green onions and mix the artichokes carefully with the help of the hands.
6. Then put all the ingredients except the lemon halves in the 2 plastic zip lock bags.
7. Seal the plastic bags and put them in the preheated to 195 F Sous Vide water bath.
8. Cook the artichokes for 2 hours.
9. Meanwhile, make the artichoke sauce: combine the garlic sauce and mustard together. Mix the mixture up.
10. Preheat the grill to 370 F.
11. When the artichokes are cooked – discard them from the sealed plastic bags and put the artichokes on the grill.
12. Cook the vegetables for 1 minute from each side.

13. Then put the prepared side dish on the serving plates.
14. Sprinkle the artichokes with the sauce and serve.
15. Enjoy!

Nutrition: calories 199, fat 11.9, fiber 6, carbs 22, protein 5

Creamy Mashed Potato

Prep time: 15 minutes
Cooking time: 2 hours
Servings: 8

Ingredients

½ cup cream
2-pound potato
1 teaspoon salt
2 tablespoon butter
2 tablespoon chives
1 teaspoon ground turmeric
½ cup fresh dill, chopped

Directions:

1. Peel the potatoes and chop them.
2. Put the chopped potatoes in the plastic Sous Vide bag and add the salt, chives, chopped dill, and ground turmeric.
3. After this, add butter and cream.
4. Seal the Sous Vide plastic bag.
5. Set the Sous Vide machine to 195 F.
6. Put the sealed plastic bag with the potato mixture in the Sous Vide machine and cook it for 2 hours.
7. After this, remove the plastic bag from the Sous Vide machine.
8. Put the potato mixture in the big bowl and blend it carefully with the help of the hand blender.
9. When the potato mixture is very smooth – the mashed potato is cooked.
10. Serve it immediately!

Nutrition: calories 144, fat 5.9, fiber 3, carbs 20.69, protein 3

Sous Vide Brussel Sprouts

Prep time: 20 minutes
Cooking time: 1.5 hours
Servings: 4

Ingredients

3 tablespoon lime juice
1 teaspoon lime zest
1-pound Brussel sprouts
1 teaspoon salt
1 teaspoon ground paprika
1 tablespoon sour cream
1 tablespoon olive oil
3 tablespoon Dijon Mustard

Directions:

1. Wash the Brussel sprouts carefully and put them in the plastic bag.
2. Add the lime zest, salt, ground paprika, and sour cream.
3. Close the plastic bag and shake it until the mixture is homogenous.
4. Then set the Sous Vide machine to 191 F.
5. Seal the plastic bag with the Brussel sprout mixture and put it in the Sous Vide machine.
6. Cook the side dish for 1.5 hours.
7. Meanwhile, preheat the grill to 400 F.
8. When the Brussel sprouts are cooked – toss them on the grill and grill for 7 minutes.
9. Stir it frequently.
10. Then sprinkle the cooked Brussel sprouts with Dijon mustard and transfer to the serving plates.

Nutrition: calories 94, fat 4.5, fiber 5, carbs 12, protein 5

Butter Sweet Corn

Prep time: 10 minutes
Cooking time: 40 minutes
Servings: 4

Ingredients

4 sweet corn on the cob
4 teaspoon white sugar
1 tablespoon turmeric
4 teaspoon butter
4 tablespoon heavy cream
1 teaspoon salt

Directions:

1. Combine the white sugar, turmeric, heavy cream, and salt in the bowl.
2. Whisk the mixture carefully.
3. After this, put the corn in the 4 plastic bags and add the whisked cream mixture.
4. Then seal the plastic bags.
5. Preheat the Sous Vide water bath to 190 F and put the sealed bags with the corn there.
6. Cook the sweet corn for 40 minutes.
7. When the dish is cooked – discard it from the sealed bags and rub with the butter.
8. Serve the corn only hot.
9. Enjoy!

Nutrition: calories 187, fat 11.4, fiber 3, carbs 21, protein 4

Green Peas with Onions

Prep time: 10 minutes
Cooking time: 2 hours
Servings: 5

Ingredients

1 cup onion
4 cup green peas
1 teaspoon sugar
½ teaspoon salt
4 tablespoon sour cream
3 tablespoon chicken stock
1 teaspoon curry
¼ teaspoon canola oil

Directions:

1. Chop the onion and combine it with the green peas.
2. Put the vegetable mixture in the plastic zip lock bag.
3. Add salt, sugar, sour cream, chicken stock, curry, and canola oil.
4. Seal the plastic bag.
5. Set Sous Vide water bath to 190 F.
6. Put the sealed plastic bag with the green peas mixture in the Sous Vide water bath and cook it for 2 hours.
7. When the time is over – transfer the content of the sealed bag directly in the serving plates.
8. Enjoy!

Nutrition: calories 126, fat 2.5, fiber 8, carbs 20, protein 7

Butter Grits

Prep time: 8 minutes
Cooking time: 3 hours
Servings: 4

Ingredients

4 tablespoon butter
10 oz. grits
10 oz. water
1 teaspoon salt
1 teaspoon ground paprika

Directions:

1. Put the grits in the plastic bag.
2. Add water, butter, salt, and ground paprika.
3. Then seal the plastic bag.
4. Put the sealed plastic bag in the preheated to 181 F Sous Vide water bath.
5. Cook the grits for 3 hours.
6. When the time is over – discard the content of the sealed bag in the serving bowls.
7. Enjoy the side dish immediately!

Nutrition: calories 173, fat 14.9, fiber 1, carbs 10, protein 1

Snacks and Appetizers

Chicken Mini Burgers

Prep time: 20 minutes
Cooking time: 30 minutes
Servings: 8

Ingredients:

1-pound ground chicken
1 teaspoon paprika
2 teaspoon ground black pepper
1 onion
1 teaspoon garlic powder
1 egg
1 teaspoon salt

Directions:

1. Put the ground chicken in the big bowl.
2. Peel the onion and grate it.
3. Beat the egg in the ground chicken mixture and add the garlic powder.
4. After this, add the grated onion and mix the meat mixture very carefully with the help of the hands.
5. After this, make 8 small burgers.
6. Sprinkle the mini burgers with the paprika, salt, and ground black pepper.
7. Then put the mini burgers in the single plastic bags and seal them.
8. Preheat the Sous Vide water bath to 133 F and put the sealed plastic bags there.
9. Cook the dish for 30 minutes.
10. Meanwhile, preheat the grill.
11. When the time is over – remove the burgers from the water bath and discard them from the plastic bags.
12. Then transfer the mini burgers on the preheated grill.
13. Roast the burgers for 2 minutes on the each side.
14. Serve the dish hot!

Nutrition: calories 109, fat 5.9, fiber 1, carbs 2.94, protein 11

French Fries

Prep time: 20 minutes
Cooking time: 25 minutes
Servings: 12

Ingredients:

3-pound potato
2 tablespoon salt
5 cup water
¼ teaspoon baking soda
1 teaspoon ground black pepper
1 cup oil, for frying

Directions:

1. Peel the potatoes and slice them into the French fries shape.
2. Preheat Sous Vide water bath to 194 F.
3. Pour water into the saucepan.
4. Add salt and baking soda and mix it well till the baking soda and salt is dissolved.
5. After this, put the prepared sliced potatoes there.
6. Stir the mixture and pour it in the plastic bag.
7. Seal the plastic bag and put it in the preheated water bath and cook it for25 minutes.
8. Meanwhile, pour the oil into the saucepan and reheat it.
9. When the time is over – remove the potatoes from the brine and dry it little with the help of the paper towel.
10. Then toss the potato in the preheated oil.
11. Cook the potato fries for 5 minutes. Stir them gently with the help of the spatula to make the potato color golden from all sides.
12. Then transfer French fries in the serving plate.
13. Sprinkle the dish with the ground black pepper.
14. Enjoy!

Nutrition: calories 89, fat 0.1, fiber 3, carbs 20, protein 2

Sweet Duck Wings

Prep time: 10 minutes
Cooking time: 7 hours
Servings: 7

Ingredients:

2-pound duck wings
1 tablespoon maple syrup
2 tablespoon sugar
1 tablespoon tomato paste
1 teaspoon salt
1 teaspoon ground black pepper
3 tablespoon butter

Directions:

1. Combine the maple syrup, sugar, tomato paste, salt, ground black pepper, and butter in the big bowl.
2. Churn the mixture well until you get the homogeneous texture and the sugar is dissolved.
3. Then put the duck wings in the plastic bag.
4. Add the churned sugar mixture and close the plastic bag.
5. Shake the plastic bag to make the mixture homogeneous.
6. Then seal the plastic bag.
7. Preheat Sous Vide water bath to 174 F.
8. Cook the wings for 7 hours.
9. When the time is over – transfer the cooked duck wings immediately in the serving bowls.
10. Enjoy!

Nutrition: calories 173, fat 5.5, fiber 0, carbs 5.24, protein 26

Baby Back Ribs

Prep time: 15 minutes
Cooking time: 12 hours
Servings: 10

Ingredients:

16 oz. pork ribs
1 tablespoon paprika
1 teaspoon salt
1 tablespoon olive oil
1 teaspoon cayenne pepper
½ tablespoon fresh rosemary
1 teaspoon ground black pepper
3 tablespoon butter
2 teaspoon apple cider vinegar
1 teaspoon hot sauce

Directions:

1. Combine the paprika, salt, cayenne pepper, fresh rosemary, and ground black pepper together. Stir the mixture with the help of the fork.
2. After this, rub the pork ribs with the spice mixture.
3. Combine the hot sauce, apple cider vinegar, and olive oil together. Whisk the mixture.
4. Then brush the pork ribs with the hot sauce mixture.
5. Put the pork ribs in the plastic bag and seal it.
6. Preheat Sous Vide water bath to 165 F and put the sealed bag there.
7. Cook the dish for 12 hours.
8. When the ribs are cooked – you can serve them immediately or bake for 10 minutes in the preheated to 365 F oven.

Nutrition: calories 111, fat 7.5, fiber 0, carbs 1.04, protein 10

Chili Chicken Wings

Prep time: 15 minutes
Cooking time: 2 hours
Servings: 8

Ingredients:

1 tablespoon chili pepper
2 teaspoon hot sauce
1 tablespoon sour cream
1 teaspoon soy sauce
1 teaspoon salt
1 teaspoon sugar
2-pound chicken wings
1 teaspoon minced garlic
2 tablespoon butter

Directions:

1. Put the chili pepper, hot sauce, sour cream, soy sauce, salt, sugar, minced garlic, and butter in the plastic zipper-lock bag.
2. Close it and shake well.
3. Then open the zipper-lock bag and add the chicken wings there.
4. Close the zipper-lock bag and shake it one more time.
5. After this, seal the plastic bag.
6. Prepare Sous Vide water bath and preheat it to 148 F.
7. Put the sealed plastic bag with the chicken wings in the water bath and cook it for 2 hours.
8. When the chicken wings are cooked – serve them immediately.
9. Enjoy!

Nutrition: calories 176, fat 7.2, fiber 0, carbs 1.25, protein 25

Sous Vide Steak Strips

Prep time: 15 minutes
Cooking time: 120 minutes
Servings: 4

Ingredients:

1-pound beef steak
1 teaspoon salt
1 teaspoon ground black pepper
½ teaspoon bay leaf
1 teaspoon turmeric
1 teaspoon thyme
5 tablespoon olive oil
1 teaspoon ground coriander
2 teaspoon butter

Directions:

1. Sprinkle the beef steak with the salt, ground black pepper, bay leaf, turmeric, thyme, and ground coriander from the both sides.
2. Then put the beef steak in the plastic bag.
3. Add butter and seal the plastic bag.
4. After this, put the sealed plastic bag in the preheated to 129 F water bath and set the timer to 120 minutes.
5. Cook the steak.
6. Meanwhile, preheat the olive oil in the skillet.
7. When the steak is cooked – toss it in the hot olive oil and roast it for 2 minutes from the each side on the medium heat.
8. Cut the cooked steak into the strips.
9. Enjoy the snack immediately!

Nutrition: calories 332, fat 25.1, fiber 0, carbs 2, protein 24

Appetizer Shrimps

Prep time: 10 minutes
Cooking time: 1 hour
Servings: 8

Ingredients:

½ cup fresh parsley
3 tablespoon fresh lemon juice
1-pound shrimps
1 teaspoon salt
1 teaspoon ground white pepper
½ teaspoon ground celery
3 tablespoon sesame oil

Directions:

1. Peel the shrimps and put them in Sous Vide plastic bag.
2. Chop the fresh parsley and add it in the plastic bag too.
3. After this, add the fresh lemon juice and salt.
4. Sprinkle the shrimps with the ground white pepper, ground celery, and sesame oil.
5. Close the plastic bag and shake it gently.
6. Then seal the plastic bag.
7. Preheat Sous Vide water bath to 140 F and put the shrimps there.
8. Cook the shrimps for 1 hour.
9. After this, discard the shrimps from the plastic bag and transfer in the serving plate.
10. Enjoy!

Nutrition: calories 107, fat 5.9, fiber 0, carbs 1.17, protein 12

Cocktail Quail Legs

Prep time: 15 minutes
Cooking time: 7 hours
Servings: 7

Ingredients:

4 tablespoon olive oil
14 oz. quail legs
1 teaspoon thyme
1 tablespoon ground coriander
1 teaspoon salt
½ tablespoon butter
1 teaspoon minced garlic

Directions:

1. Put the quail legs in the plate in the single layer.
2. Then sprinkle the poultry with the thyme, ground coriander, salt, and minced garlic.
3. Massage the quail legs with the help of the hands gently and transfer them to the plastic bag in a single layer.
4. Then add the butter and seal the plastic bag.
5. Preheat the water bath to 143 F and cook the quail legs for 7 hours.
6. When the dish is cooked – transfer it to the cocktail plate and serve.
7. Enjoy!

Nutrition: calories 152, fat 11.1, fiber 0, carbs 0, protein 12

Deviled Eggs

Prep time: 10 minutes
Cooking time: 1 hour
Servings: 14

Ingredients:

7 eggs
1 tablespoon paprika
1 teaspoon salt
1 tablespoon mustard
2 teaspoon mayo sauce
1 teaspoon cayenne pepper

Directions:

1. Set Sous Vide water bath to 170 F and put the eggs there.
2. Cook the eggs for 1 hour.
3. Meanwhile, combine the salt, mustard, mayo sauce, and cayenne pepper in the bowl.
4. Mix the mixture.
5. When the eggs are cooked – chill them well using the ice bath.
6. Then peel the eggs and cut them into the halves.
7. Remove the egg yolks and blend them till you get the smooth texture. Use the hand blender.
8. After this, combine the egg mixture with the mayo sauce mixture and mix it.
9. Fill the egg whites with the smooth mixture.
10. Enjoy!

Nutrition: calories 67, fat 4.9, fiber 0, carbs 1, protein 5

Veggie Bundles

Prep time: 20 minutes
Cooking time: 30 minutes
Servings: 4

Ingredients:

2 sweet pepper
1 zucchini
1 teaspoon salt
1 teaspoon paprika
1 eggplant
2 tablespoon olive oil
1 teaspoon ground black pepper
1 teaspoon garlic powder

Directions:

1. Discard the seeds from the sweet peppers.
2. Cut the sweet peppers and eggplant into the thick strips.
3. After this, sprinkle the vegetable strips with the salt, paprika, ground black pepper, and garlic powder.
4. Separate the vegetable strips into 4 parts.
5. Then slice the wide ribbons from the zucchini and wrap the strips parts in the zucchini ribbons.
6. Put the vegetable bundles in the plastic bag and seal it.
7. Cook the veggie bundles at 183 F for 30 minutes.
8. When the veggie bundles are cooked – remove them gently from the plastic bag and serve.
9. Enjoy!

Nutrition: calories 128, fat 7.3, fiber 5, carbs 15.96, protein 3

Fish and Seafood

Rosemary Salmon Fillet

Prep time: 15 minutes
Cooking time: 40 minutes
Servings: 6

Ingredients:

½ lime
1 tablespoon vinegar
2 tablespoon canola oil
1 teaspoon oregano
1 teaspoon turmeric
1 tablespoon salt
3 oz. fresh rosemary
2-pound salmon fillet
¼ cup cherry tomatoes

Directions:

1. Slice the lime.
2. Combine the canola oil, oregano, turmeric, salt, and fresh rosemary in the bowl.
3. Mix the mixture up.
4. After this, brush the salmon with the spice mixture and put it in the Sous Vide plastic bag.
5. Add the sliced lime and close the plastic bag.
6. Seal the plastic bag using the vacuum method.
7. Then set Sous Vide water bath to 167 F and place the salmon there.
8. Cook the salmon fillet for 40 minutes.
9. When the salmon is cooked – remove it from the plastic bag and discard the sliced lime.
10. Serve it!

Nutrition: calories 295, fat 16.4, fiber 2, carbs 3.77, protein 32

Hot Royal Shrimps

Prep time: 25 minutes
Cooking time: 35 minutes
Servings: 5

Ingredients:

2 tablespoon hot sauce
17 oz. Royal shrimps
1 tablespoon salt
3 tablespoon lemon juice
2 tablespoon butter
1 tablespoon cayenne pepper
1 teaspoon chili flakes

Directions:

1. Peel the royal shrimps.
2. Then whisk together the hot sauce, salt, lemon juice, cayenne pepper, and chili flakes.
3. Sprinkle the royal shrimps with the hot sauce mixture and leave it for 15 minutes to marinate.
4. Then put the shrimps in the plastic bag.
5. Add the remaining hot sauce mixture and butter.
6. After this, close the plastic bag and seal it.
7. Set Sous Vide water bath to 149 F and preheat it.
8. Put the shrimps in the preheated Sous Vide bath and cook it for 35 minutes.
9. When the royal shrimps are cooked – chill them in the ice bath well and then discard from the sealed plastic bag.
10. Enjoy!

Nutrition: calories 130, fat 5.4, fiber 1, carbs 1.6, protein 20

Wasabi Shrimp Tails

Prep time: 20 minutes
Cooking time: 30 minutes
Servings: 4

Ingredients:

14 oz. shrimps
3 tablespoon wasabi
¼ cup butter
1 tablespoon rosemary
1 teaspoon dried dill
1 tablespoon ground paprika
1 teaspoon oregano
2 teaspoon lemon juice
1 tablespoon heavy cream

Directions:

1. Peel the shrimps and cut the tails. Then put them in the zipper-lock bag.
2. Add the butter, wasabi, rosemary, dried dill, ground paprika, oregano, and lemon juice.
3. Close the zipper-lock bag and shake it well.
4. Then seal the zipper-lock bag and massage the shrimps gently.
5. Set Sous Vide water bath to 147 F and put the sealed shrimps.
6. Cook the shrimps for 30 minutes.
7. Meanwhile, preheat the heavy cream until it is hot.
8. When the shrimp tails are cooked – transfer them to the appetizer bowl and sprinkle with the hot heavy cream.
9. Serve it!

Nutrition: calories 222, fat 14.6, fiber 1, carbs 1.76, protein 21

Delightful Octopus

Prep time: 10 minutes
Cooking time: 4 hours
Servings: 4

Ingredients:

9 oz. octopus
3 tablespoon olive oil
1 teaspoon salt
1 tablespoon ground black pepper
1 teaspoon minced garlic
2 tablespoon lemon zest
1 tablespoon vinegar

Directions:

1. Combine the salt, olive oil, ground black pepper, minced garlic, lemon zest, and vinegar in the bowl.
2. Whisk the mixture.
3. Then chop the octopus in the medium pieces and put it in the Sous Vide plastic bag.
4. Add the whisked oily mixture and close the plastic bag.
5. Seal the plastic bag.
6. Set Sous Vide water bath to 180 F.
7. When the water bath is preheated – put the sealed plastic bag with the octopus there.
8. Cook the octopus for 4 hours.
9. When the octopus is cooked – chill it using the ice bath.
10. Then discard the octopus from the sealed plastic bag and serve it.
11. Enjoy!

Nutrition: calories 150, fat 10.8, fiber 0, carbs 3.26, protein 10

Savory Halibut

Prep time: 20 minutes
Cooking time: 45 minutes
Servings: 6

Ingredients:

1 tablespoon fresh ginger
1 teaspoon oregano
1 teaspoon ground white pepper
1 teaspoon paprika
½ teaspoon soy sauce
1 teaspoon chili flakes
½ cup fresh basil
¼ lemon
3 tablespoon butter
2-pound halibut

Directions:
1. Grate the fresh ginger and combine it with oregano, ground white pepper, and paprika, soy sauce, and chili flakes.
2. Whisk the mixture.
3. Slice the lemon.
4. Brush the halibut with the fresh ginger mixture.
5. Then put the sliced lemon over the halibut.
6. Wrap the halibut in the fresh basil and put it in the plastic bag. Seal the plastic bag.
7. Preheat the Sous Vide water bath to 142 F and put the halibut there.
8. Cook the fish for 45 minutes.
9. When the halibut is cooked – discard it from the water bath and they remove it from the sealed bag.
10. Then discard the lemon and the basil.

Nutrition: calories 341, fat 26.9, fiber 1, carbs 1.74, protein 22

Pickled Shrimps

Prep time: 15 minutes
Cooking time: 30 minutes
Servings: 8

Ingredients:

1 tablespoon fennel seeds
1 teaspoon coriander seeds
1 teaspoon thyme
1 teaspoon cilantro
½ teaspoon oregano
½ tablespoon mustard seeds
2 tablespoon olive oil
1 teaspoon lemon zest
1-pound shrimps
2 oz. garlic cloves, peeled
1 tablespoon bay leaf
3 tablespoon vinegar
¼ cup lime juice
1 white onion
1 teaspoon salt

Directions:

1. Peel the onion and grate it.
2. Combine the grated onion, lemon zest, lime juice, and vinegar together in the Sous Vide plastic bag.
3. Peel the shrimps and add them in the plastic bag too.
4. After this, add the fennel seeds, coriander seeds, thyme, cilantro, oregano, mustard seeds, salt, and olive oil.
5. Close the Sous Vide plastic bag and shake it.
6. Then seal the plastic bag using the vacuum technique.
7. Set the Sous Vide machine to 149 F and cook the shrimps for 30 minutes.

8. When the pickled shrimps are cooked – transfer them to the glass jar and close the lid.
9. Serve the pickled shrimps chilled and keep them in the fridge.
10. Enjoy!

Nutrition: calories 120, fat 4.5, fiber 1, carbs 7, protein 13

Trout in Coconut Sauce

Prep time: 20 minutes
Cooking time: 30 minutes
Servings: 4

Ingredients:

1-pound trout
1 cup coconut milk
1 teaspoon salt
1 teaspoon ground black pepper
½ teaspoon chipotle
1 oz. kaffir leaves
2 teaspoon fish sauce
¼ cup chicken stock
1 teaspoon sugar
1 teaspoon lemon juice
1 teaspoon ground black pepper
3 tablespoon fresh cilantro
1 tablespoon olive oil

Directions:

1. Sprinkle the trout with the ground black pepper and salt.
2. Put the fish in the plastic bag and close it.
3. Seal the plastic bag.
4. Set Sous Vide water bath to 131 F and cook the fish for 15 minutes.
5. Meanwhile, combine the coconut milk, salt, ground black pepper, chipotle, kaffir leaves, fish sauce, chicken stock, sugar, and lemon juice, 1 teaspoon of ground black pepper, fresh cilantro, and olive oil.
6. Stir the mixture.
7. Pour the liquid mixture into the saucepan and reheat it until it starts to boil.

8. When the time is over – remove the fish from the plastic bag.
9. Then pour the prepared sauce in the plastic bag.
10. Add the trout and seal it.
11. Put the fish in the water bath and boil it at 131 F for 15 minutes more.
12. Then transfer the fish to the serving plates.
13. Sprinkle it with the sauce.
14. Enjoy!

Nutrition: calories 359, fat 25.5, fiber 2, carbs 7.46, protein 27

Thai Calamari

Prep time: 18 minutes
Cooking time: 2 hours
Servings: 5

Ingredients:

17 oz. calamari tubes
1 teaspoon salt
½ teaspoon red pepper
7 oz. pineapple chunks
1 teaspoon chili sauce
1 teaspoon sour-sweet sauce
1 teaspoon butter
2 teaspoon turmeric

Directions:

1. Peel the calamari tubes and chop them roughly.
2. Sprinkle the chopped calamari with the salt, red pepper, chili sauce, sour-sweet sauce, and turmeric.
3. Mix it gently and put in the plastic bag.
4. Set Sous Vide water bath to 136 F and preheat it.
5. Put the pineapple chunks in the plastic bag too.
6. Add butter and close it.
7. Then seal the plastic bag and put it in the water bath.
8. Cook Thai Calamari for 2 hours.
9. When the dish is cooked – transfer it with all the liquid and pineapple chunks in the bowl.
10. Enjoy the dish immediately!

Nutrition: calories 224, fat 3.5, fiber 1, carbs 16.22, protein 30

Sous Vide Seabass

Prep time: 15 minutes
Cooking time: 70 minutes
Servings: 4

Ingredients:

4 tablespoon pineapple juice
1 tablespoon lemon juice
3 tablespoon orange juice
1 teaspoon salt
1 teaspoon sugar
2 teaspoon ground white pepper
1-pound sea bass fillet
2 teaspoon thyme
½ teaspoon basil
1 tablespoon olive oil
1 teaspoon garlic, sliced

Directions:

1. Cut the sea bass fillet into 4 parts and put the fish in the plastic bag.
2. Add the lemon juice, orange juice, salt, sugar, ground white pepper, and thyme.
3. Then add the basil, olive oil, and sliced garlic.
4. Close the plastic bag and seal it.
5. Set Sous Vide water bath equipment to 132 F and put the prepared sealed bag there.
6. Cook the fish for 70 minutes.
7. When the fish is cooked – transfer it to the serving plates.
8. Sprinkle the fish with the remaining sauce gently.
9. Enjoy!

Nutrition: calories 168, fat 5.7, fiber 1, carbs 6.75, protein 22

Cinnamon Haddock

Prep time: 15 minutes
Cooking time: 42 minutes
Servings: 7

Ingredients:

21 oz. haddock fillet
1 tablespoon tomato sauce
1 tablespoon sour cream
1 teaspoon salt
2 teaspoon ground cinnamon
1 red onion
2 teaspoon sesame oil
1 tablespoon sesame seeds
1 teaspoon lemongrass
1 teaspoon rice vinegar

Directions:

1. Brush the haddock with the tomato sauce, sour cream, and sesame oil.
2. After this, sprinkle the fish with the salt, ground cinnamon, lemongrass, and sesame seeds from the each side.
3. After this, sprinkle the fish with the rice vinegar.
4. Chop the red onion and put it in the Sous Vide plastic bag.
5. Then add the prepared haddock and close the plastic bag.
6. Seal the plastic bag using the vacuum method.
7. Set Sous Vide water bath to 143 F and put the sealed haddock there.
8. Cook the fish for 42 minutes.
9. When the time is over – discard the haddock from the water bath and separate it into 7 parts.

10. Sprinkle every piece of the haddock with the cooked chopped onion.
11. Enjoy!

Nutrition: calories 95, fat 2.6, fiber 1, carbs 2.81, protein 14

Lemon Seabass

Prep time: 15 minutes
Cooking time: 30 minutes
Servings: 4

Ingredients:

1 lemon
2-pound sea bass fillet
1 teaspoon ground white pepper
1 teaspoon salt
4 tablespoon butter
1 tablespoon cream
1 teaspoon dried garlic

Directions:

1. Grate the lemon zest and chop the lemon flesh.
2. Then combine the ground white pepper, salt, and fried garlic in the bowl. Stir the mixture.
3. Rub the seabass fillet with the ground white mixture and add the lemon zest.
4. Then churn the cream, butter, and lemon flesh until it is smooth.
5. Brush the seabass fillet with the churned mixture and put the fish in the plastic Sous Vide bag.
6. Seal the bag.
7. Set the Sous Vide water bath to 136 F and put the sealed seabass fillet there.
8. Cook the seabass fillet for 30 minutes.
9. When the fish is cooked – remove it from the plastic bag and cut into 4 pieces.
10. Serve the fish immediately.

Nutrition: calories 503, fat 3.6, fiber 1.7, carbs 2.3, protein 50.8

Poultry

Honey Duck Breast

Prep time: 10 minutes
Cooking time: 60 minutes
Servings: 4

Ingredients:

1-pound duck breast
2 tablespoon honey
1 teaspoon salt
1 teaspoon thyme
1 teaspoon cilantro
1 teaspoon oregano
½ teaspoon paprika
1 teaspoon garlic sauce
1 tablespoon sesame oil

Directions:

1. Cut the duck breast into 2 parts.
2. After this, combine the honey, salt, thyme, cilantro, oregano, paprika, and sesame oil in the bowl.
3. Whisk it until the mixture is homogenous.
4. After this, add the garlic sauce and continue to whisk the mixture until it is smooth.
5. Then brush the duck breasts with the prepared garlic sauce mixture generously.
6. Preheat Sous Vide water bath to 158 F.
7. Then put the chicken breasts in the plastic bag.
8. Add the remaining garlic sauce mixture and close the plastic bag. Massage it gently.
9. Then seal the plastic bag and put it in the preheated water bath.
10. Cook the duck breasts for 60 minutes.
11. When the time is over – remove the duck breasts from the plastic bag and separate them into 4 parts.
12. Serve the dish!

Nutrition: calories 203, fat 8.3, fiber 0, carbs 9, protein 23

Sous Vide Chocolate Grilled Chicken

Prep time: 20 minutes
Cooking time: 54 minutes
Servings: 5

Ingredients:

2 oz milk chocolate
2 tablespoon butter
1 tablespoon heavy cream
1 teaspoon ground coriander
1 teaspoon ground ginger
1 teaspoon ground black pepper
½ teaspoon salt
1 teaspoon balsamic vinegar
14 oz chicken breast
1 teaspoon garlic, sliced
1 tablespoon sunflower oil

Directions:

1. Crush the milk chocolate and put it in the bowl. Add the butter.
2. Melt the mixture and whisk it to make homogenous.
3. After this, add the heavy cream and mix it up well again.
4. Then add the ground coriander, ground ginger, ground black pepper, salt, balsamic vinegar, and mix it well with the help of the fork.
5. Add sliced garlic and mix it up.
6. After this, put the chicken breast in the plastic bag.
7. Add the chocolate mixture and close the plastic bag.
8. Shake it well to combine the chicken breast and the chocolate mixture well.
9. Seal the plastic bag and put it in the preheated to 149 F Sous Vide water bath.
10. Cook the chicken breast for 54 minutes.

11. Meanwhile, preheat the grill and brush it with the sunflower oil.
12. When the chicken breast is cooked – remove it from the plastic bag and transfer to the grill.
13. Grill the poultry for 3 minutes from the each side or till you get the light golden color of the chicken sides.
14. After this, slice the chicken breast and serve it immediately.
15. Enjoy!

Nutrition: calories 230, fat 16.3, fiber 0, carbs 3, protein 17

Herbed Chicken Drumsticks

Prep time: 20 minutes
Cooking time: 57 minutes
Servings: 7

Ingredients:

1 tablespoon kaffir lime leaves
2 tablespoon fresh coriander leaves
1 teaspoon thyme
1 teaspoon ground white pepper
½ teaspoon cinnamon
1 teaspoon dried mint
1 teaspoon salt
16 oz chicken drumsticks
1 tablespoon olive oil

Directions:

1. Chop the kaffir lime leaves and fresh coriander leaves.
2. Combine the leaves with the thyme, ground white pepper, cinnamon, dried mint, and salt.
3. Mix the mixture with the help of the hands.
4. After this, put the chicken drumsticks in the big mixing bowl.
5. Sprinkle the chicken with the leaves mixture and stir it carefully.
6. After this, add the olive oil and mix it up with the help of the fingertips.
7. Then leave the chicken drumsticks for 20 minutes to marinate in the cold place (fridge).
8. Meanwhile, preheat Sous Vide water bath to 153 F.
9. When the time is over – transfer the chicken drumsticks in the plastic bag and seal it.
10. Put the sealed plastic bag in the preheated water bath and cook the dish for 57 minutes.

11. When the chicken drumsticks are cooked – discard them from the plastic bag and dry gently with the help of the paper towel.
12. Then transfer the cooked dish to the serving plates and serve the dish warm.
13. Enjoy!

Nutrition: calories 125, fat 7.9, fiber 0, carbs 1, protein 12

Chicken Tights with Dried Tomatoes

Prep time: 15 minutes
Cooking time: 60 minutes
Servings: 7

Ingredients:

1 egg
3 oz dried tomatoes
1 tablespoon palm sugar
1 teaspoon thyme
1 teaspoon coriander seeds
2 tablespoon olive oil
1 yellow onion
1 teaspoon salt
2-pound chicken tights
1/3 teaspoon fresh rosemary

Directions:

1. Crack the egg into the bowl and whisk it with the help of the hand whisker.
2. After this, sprinkle the whisked egg with the palm sugar, thyme, coriander seeds, salt, and fresh rosemary.
3. Peel the yellow onion and slice it.
4. Put the sliced onion in the plastic bag.
5. Add the olive oil and chicken tights.
6. After this, whisk the egg mixture again and pour it into the plastic bag.
7. Then slice the dried tomatoes and add them in the plastic bag too.
8. Then close the plastic bag and seal it.
9. Massage the plastic bag to get the homogeneous chicken tights mass.
10. Preheat Sous Vide water bath to 149 F and put the sealed chicken tights there.
11. Cook the chicken tights for 60 minutes.

12. When the time is over – remove the chicken from the water bath and discard from the plastic bag.
13. Serve the chicken tights with all the content of the plastic bag.
14. Enjoy!

Nutrition: calories 210, fat 8.8, fiber 1, carbs 3, protein 28

Sous Vide Teriyaki Duck Strips

Prep time: 15 minutes
Cooking time: 54 minutes
Servings: 8

Ingredients:

17 oz duck fillet
4 tablespoon teriyaki sauce
3 garlic cloves, minced
1 teaspoon salt
1 teaspoon ground black pepper
1 teaspoon cilantro
1 teaspoon oregano
1 tablespoon olive oil

Directions:

1. Combine the teriyaki sauce and minced garlic together in the mixing bowl.
2. Add the salt, ground black pepper, cilantro, and oregano. Mix it up.
3. Cut the duck fillet into the strips and sprinkle them with the teriyaki sauce mixture.
4. Then put the duck strips in the plastic zip lock bag and close it.
5. Seal the plastic zip lock bag.
6. Set Sous Vide water bath to 160 F and put the prepared plastic bag there.
7. Cook the duck strips for 54 minutes.
8. After this, sprinkle the skillet with the olive oil and preheat it well.
9. When the duck strips are cooked – transfer them to the preheated skillet and fry for 5 minutes on the medium heat. Stir it frequently.
10. Then transfer the prepared duck strips in the plates and serve.

11. Enjoy!

Nutrition: calories 154, fat 10.9, fiber 0, carbs 2, protein 11

Tender Chicken Skin Balls

Prep time: 20 minutes
Cooking time: 2 hours
Servings: 5

Ingredients:

6 oz ground pork
8 oz chicken skin
1 tablespoon paprika
1 egg
¼ cup fresh dill
1 teaspoon ground black pepper
1 teaspoon onion powder
1 teaspoon olive oil
2 teaspoon turmeric

Directions:

1. Put the ground pork in the bowl and add the paprika, and ground black pepper.
2. After this, sprinkle the ground pork with the onion powder and turmeric.
3. Crack the egg in the ground pork mixture and stir it carefully with the help of the spoon.
4. Then wash the fresh dill and chop it.
5. Add the chopped dill to the ground pork mixture and stir it carefully again.
6. Then separate the chicken skin into 5 parts and put the ground pork mixture in every part.
7. Wrap the chicken skin and secure it with the thread.
8. Then put every chicken skin ball in the plastic bag and seal the plastic bag,
9. Put the plastic bag in the preheated to 152 F Sous Vide water bath.
10. Cook the dish for 2 hours.

11. When the time is over – pour the olive oil in the skillet and make it hot.
12. Transfer the content of the plastic bag in the hot oil and fry it till you get the golden sides of the chicken skin balls.
13. After this, dry the cooked dish with the paper towel and serve them.
14. Enjoy!

Nutrition: calories 228, fat 14.7, fiber 1, carbs 3, protein 21

Chicken Fillet with Cream Mushroom Sauce

Prep time: 25 minutes
Cooking time: 95 minutes
Servings: 4

Ingredients:

2-pound chicken fillet
1 teaspoon salt
1 teaspoon ground black pepper
1 teaspoon curry powder
8 oz mushrooms
½ cup cream
2 tablespoon flour
1 teaspoon cilantro
1 onion, peeled
1 teaspoon ground white pepper
1 carrot, peeled
2 teaspoon sesame oil
1 teaspoon olive oil

Directions:

1. Cut the chicken fillet into 4 parts.
2. Then sprinkle every chicken part with the salt, ground black pepper, and curry powder.
3. Mix the chicken fillets with the help of the hands.
4. Then put the chicken fillets in the plastic bag and seal it.
5. Cook the sealed chicken fillets at the preheated to 140 F water bath for 95 minutes.
6. Meanwhile, cook the sauce: Wash the mushrooms and slice them.
7. Then slice the onion and carrot.
8. After this, toss the sliced vegetables in the saucepan and add the sesame oil.

9. Roast the vegetables on the medium heat and stir it with the help of the wooden spatula frequently.
10. After 3 minutes, add the ground white pepper and cream.
11. Mix the sauce carefully and add the flour.
12. Then mix the sauce until it smooth and cook it on the medium heat for 3 minutes more or till it is thick.
13. When the sauce is cooked – let it chill little.
14. Transfer the cooked chicken fillets in the serving plates.
15. Then sprinkle the mushroom sauce over every chicken fillet generously.
16. Serve the prepared dish immediately.
17. Enjoy!

Nutrition: calories 858, fat 79.1, fiber 1, carbs 19, protein 19

Chicken Cutlets with Grated Onion Sauce

Prep time: 20 minutes
Cooking time: 45 minutes
Servings: 4

Ingredients:

3 tablespoon Dijon mustard
½ cup milk
2 yellow onion, peeled
1 teaspoon salt
2 tablespoons cornstarch
1 tablespoons corn flour
1 teaspoon ground black pepper
1-pound chicken cutlets
1 tablespoon lime zest
1 teaspoon oregano
1 teaspoon cilantro
2 teaspoon garlic powder
1 tablespoon olive oil

Directions:

1. Sprinkle the chicken cutlets with the lime zest, oregano, cilantro, and garlic powder.
2. Massage the chicken cutlets to make them soak the spices.
3. After this, sprinkle the chicken cutlets with the olive oil and put them in Sous Vide plastic bag.
4. After this, seal the plastic bag and preheat Sous Vide to 146 F.
5. Put the cutlets there and cook them for 45 minutes.
6. Meanwhile, make the onion sauce.
7. Grate the yellow onions and put them in the saucepan.
8. Add the milk and Dijon mustard. Whisk the mixture with the help of the hand whisker.

9. After this, add the salt, cornstarch, corn flour, and ground black pepper.
10. Whisk the sauce carefully and cook it on the medium heat until it starts to boil.
11. Then remove the sauce from the heat and leave it with the closed lid.
12. When the chicken cutlets are cooked – transfer them to the serving plates.
13. Then pour the onion sauce over the chicken cutlets.
14. Serve the dish hot.
15. Enjoy!

Nutrition: calories 236, fat 8, fiber 2, carbs 15, protein 26

Chicken Adobo

Prep time: 25 minutes
Cooking time: 4 hours
Servings: 6

Ingredients:

2-pound chicken tights
3 tablespoon dried bay leaf
¼ cup garlic cloves, peeled
3 tablespoon peppercorn
½ cup soy sauce
1 cup chicken stock
2 tablespoon wine vinegar

Directions:

1. Put the chicken tights in the plastic zip lock bag.
2. Then add the dried bay leaves, peppercorn, and soy sauce.
3. Crash the peeled garlic cloves and add them in the plastic bag too.
4. Close the zipper lock bag and seal it.
5. Preheat the water bath to 155 F and put the sealed bag there.
6. Cook the chicken tights for 4 hours.
7. After this, transfer the content of the sealed bag in the saucepan and start to preheat it on the medium heat.
8. Then add the wine vinegar and chicken stock.
9. Mix the chicken tights gently and close the lid.
10. Cook the chicken adobo for 10 minutes more or until the meat is cooked.
11. Serve the dish immediately.

Nutrition: calories 294, fat 12.6, fiber 1, carbs 9.49, protein 4

Chicken Tikka Masala

Prep time: 25 minutes
Cooking time: 60 minutes
Servings: 6

Ingredients:

> *1 tablespoon garam masala*
> *1 teaspoon cumin*
> *½ teaspoon ground black pepper*
> *1 teaspoon chili flakes*
> *1 teaspoon coriander*
> *¼ teaspoon ground cardamom*
> *2 tablespoons ghee*
> *1 white onion*
> *2 teaspoon olive oil*
> *¼ cup heavy cream*
> *4 tablespoon tomato paste*
> *2-pound chicken breast, skinless, boneless*

Directions:

1. Combine the garam masala, cumin, ground black pepper, chili flakes, coriander, and ground cardamom in the big bowl.
2. Mix the mixture.
3. Cut the chicken breast into the cubes and put the chicken cubes in the plastic bag.
4. Add the garam masala mixture and the ghee and close the plastic bag.
5. Then shake it to make the homogenous mass.
6. Preheat Sous Vide water bath to 162 F and put the sealed plastic bag there.
7. Cook the chicken for 60 minutes.
8. Meanwhile, chop the white onion and toss in the saucepan.

9. Add the olive oil and roast it on the medium heat for 3 minutes.
10. After this, add the heavy cream, tomato paste, and mix it up.
11. Let the mixture boils for 6 minutes on the medium heat. Stir it frequently.
12. When the chicken is cooked – transfer the content of the plastic bag in the saucepan and mix it up.
13. Cook the adobo chicken for 10 minutes more on the medium heat.
14. When the chicken adobo is cooked – serve it immediately.
15. Enjoy!

Nutrition: calories 311, fat 17.6, fiber 1, carbs 5, protein 33

Sous Vide Chicken Tacos

Prep time: 20 minutes
Cooking time: 43 minutes
Servings: 5

Ingredients:

1 avocado, pitted
13 oz chicken breast, boneless, skinless
1 teaspoon salt
1 teaspoon cilantro
1 tablespoon taco seasoning
5 corn tortillas
2 tablespoon mayo sauce
3 tablespoon lemon juice
4 oz Cheddar cheese

Directions:

1. Combine the salt, cilantro, and taco seasoning in the small mixing bowl.
2. Stir the mixture gently.
3. Then rub the chicken breast with the prepared spice mixture well.
4. Put the chicken breast in Sous Vide plastic bag and close it.
5. Then use the sealing method to vacuum the plastic bag with chicken.
6. After this, set Sous Vide water bath to 146.5 F and put the sealed plastic bag there.
7. Cook the chicken breast for 43 minutes.
8. If the chicken is not cooked enough after the time is passed – bake it for 10 minutes more at the preheated to 365 F oven.
9. Meanwhile, shed Cheddar cheese.
10. Combine the mayo sauce and lemon juice together. Whisk the sauce.

11. Then spread the corn tortillas with the mayo sauce mixture well.
12. Sprinkle the corn tortillas with the shredded cheese.
13. When the chicken is cooked – remove it from the plastic bag and shred with the help of the fork.
14. After this, sprinkle the corn tortillas with the shredded chicken breast and wrap them to make tacos.
15. Serve the dish warm.
16. Enjoy!

Nutrition: calories 293, fat 15.4, fiber 5, carbs 19, protein 21

Meat

Rosemary Pork Chop

Prep time: 12 minutes
Cooking time: 60 minutes
Servings: 4

Ingredients:

> *1-pound pork chop*
> *2 oz fresh rosemary*
> *1 teaspoon ground black pepper*
> *1 teaspoon salt*
> *1 tablespoon olive oil*
> *¼ teaspoon ground white pepper*

Directions:

1. Combine the ground black pepper, salt, and ground white pepper together in the shallow bowl.
2. Stir the spices gently with the help of the fork.
3. After this sprinkle the pork chop with the spice mixture.
4. Transfer the pork chop in the zip lock style bag.
5. Add the fresh rosemary and olive oil, and close the zip lock style bag.
6. Then seal the bag.
7. Set Sous Vide water bath to 145 F and preheat it.
8. After this, put the sealed zip lock-style bag in the water bath and cook it for 60 minutes.
9. When the pork chop is cooked – discard it from the zip lock bag and transfer to the serving plates.
10. Enjoy!

Nutrition: calories 291, fat 16.8, fiber 2, carbs 4, protein 30

Classic Pork Cutlets

Prep time: 15 minutes
Cooking time: 60 minutes
Servings: 6

Ingredients:

1 teaspoon salt
1 teaspoon ground black pepper
1 teaspoon paprika
½ cup panko bread crumbs
2-pound ground pork
1 egg
2 tablespoon butter
1 tablespoon flour

Directions:

1. Beat the egg in the mixer bowl and mix it up.
2. Then add the ground black pepper, paprika, ground pork, and flour.
3. Mix the mixture well until you get the prepared cutlet forcemeat.
4. After this, make the medium cutlets from the ground pork mixture and transfer them to the separated plastic bags.
5. Seal the plastic bags.
6. Then Set Sous Vide water bath to 141 F.
7. When the water bath is preheated – put the sealed plastic bags in the vessel and cook them for 60 minutes.
8. When the time is over – discard the cutlets from the plastic bags.
9. Preheat the skillet well and toss the butter there.
10. Sprinkle every pork cutlet with the panko bread crumbs and put them in the melted hot butter.

11. Roast the cutlets for 1 minutes on the each side or until they are golden brown.
12. Then dry the pork gently with the help of the paper towel.
13. Enjoy!

Nutrition: calories 521, fat 37, fiber 0, carbs 4, protein 41

Soft Tender Pork Ribs

Prep time: 25 minutes
Cooking time: 35 hours
Servings: 8

Ingredients:

1 teaspoon mustard seeds
1 teaspoon fennel seeds
1 teaspoon coriander seeds
2 tablespoon tomato paste
1 tablespoon olive oil
3 tablespoon garlic cloves, peeled
1 teaspoon dried dill
1 tablespoon dried thyme
1 tablespoon sugar
¼ cup soy sauce
1 teaspoon onion powder
3 tablespoon apple cider vinegar
1 tablespoon butter
21 oz pork ribs
4 tablespoon ketchup

Directions:

1. Separate the ribs into the servings and put them in the vacuum plastic bag.
2. After this, add the mustard seeds, fennel seeds, coriander seeds, olive oil, peeled garlic cloves, dried dill, dried thyme onion powder, and apple cider vinegar.
3. Add the soy sauce.
4. Close the vacuum bag and shake it gently. You can use 3 plastic bags for the pork ribs.
5. After this, seal the vacuum bag.
6. Set Sous Vide water bath to 148 F and put the sealed plastic bag there when it is preheated.

7. After this, cook the pork ribs for 35 hours.
8. Prepare the sauce for baking: combine the ketchup and tomato sauce together.
9. Mix the mixture.
10. When the pork ribs are cooked – discard them from the plastic bag and transfer in the tray.
11. Brush the pork ribs with the tomato sauce mixture well.
12. Preheat the oven to 365 F.
13. Add the butter in the tray with the pork ribs and put it in the oven.
14. Bake the pork ribs for 15 minutes.
15. When the time is over – let the pork ribs chill gently.
16. Serve it!

Nutrition: calories 183, fat 9, fiber 1, carbs 9, protein 17

Thyme Pork Tenderloin

Prep time: 15 minutes
Cooking time: 88 minutes
Servings: 5

Ingredients:

16 oz pork tenderloin
1 tablespoon curry powder
1 teaspoon salt
½ teaspoon garlic powder
½ teaspoon onion powder
2 teaspoon dried thyme
¼ cup fresh thyme leaves
1 tablespoon butter
1 teaspoon oregano
1 white onion
2 tablespoon fresh parsley chopped
1 teaspoon sunflower oil

Directions:

1. Melt butter and combine it with the sunflower oil.
2. Churn the mixture and add the dried thyme, oregano, chopped fresh parsley, and curry powder.
3. Mix it up.
4. Rub the pork tenderloin with the garlic powder, and onion powder.
5. Put the fresh thyme leaves in the vacuum plastic bag.
6. Peel the onion and chop it into 4 parts.
7. Add the chopped onion in the plastic bag.
8. After this, brush the pork tenderloin with the sunflower oil spiced mixture.
9. Put the pork tenderloin in the plastic bag and add all the remaining sunflower oil mixture.
10. After this, close the plastic bag and seal it.

11. Preheat Sous Vide water bath to 138 F and put the pork tenderloin mixture there.
12. Cook the dish for 88 minutes.
13. When the time is over – discard the meat from the water bath and transfer it to the serving plates.
14. Enjoy!

Nutrition: calories 176, fat 6.7, fiber 2, carbs 4, protein 24

Bell Pepper Pork Rolls

Prep time: 25 minutes
Cooking time: 65 minutes
Servings: 4

Ingredients:

12 oz pork fillet
2 bell peppers
1 red onion
2 tablespoon salsa
1 teaspoon salt
1 teaspoon ground black pepper
4 teaspoon butter
3 tablespoon fresh dill, chopped
1 tablespoon cream cheese

Directions:

1. Beat the pork fillet from the each side and cut it into 4 parts.
2. Then remove the seeds from the bell peppers and cut them into the strips.
3. Peel the onion and chop it.
4. Combine the bell pepper strips and chopped red onion in the bowl.
5. Sprinkle the pork fillets with the salt and ground black pepper.
6. Sprinkle the bell pepper mixture with the chopped fresh dill.
7. Combine the salsa with the cream cheese and whisk it.
8. After this, spread the pork fillets with the cream cheese mixture from the one side.
9. Add the bell pepper mixture and make the rolls.
10. Put the rolls into vacuum bags and seal the bags.
11. Set Sous Vide water bath to 146 F.

12. When the water bath is preheated – put the sealed plastic bags there.
13. Cook the pork rolls for 65 minutes.
14. When the time is over – transfer the pork rolls in the serving plates and cut every roll into 2 parts.
15. Serve it!

Nutrition: calories 314, fat 20.8, fiber 2, carbs 9, protein 24

Juicy Pork Steak

Prep time: 15 minutes
Cooking time: 55 minutes
Servings: 6

Ingredients:

1 oz dried bay leaf
1 tablespoon salt
2-pound pork steak
2 tablespoon olive oil
1 teaspoon peppercorns
½ teaspoon ground black pepper
1 teaspoon paprika
3 tablespoon dried celery

Directions:

1. Put the pork steak in the 1-gallon plastic bag.
2. Add the salt, peppercorns, ground black pepper, paprika, and dried celery.
3. After this, add bay leaf and olive oil.
4. Close the plastic bag and massage the meat to make it soak all the spices.
5. Set Sous Vide water bath to 149 F.
6. When the water bath is preheated – put the plastic bag with the pork steak there.
7. Cook the dish for 55 minutes.
8. Then preheat the skillet on the high heat.
9. When the skillet is preheated – transfer the content of the plastic bag there.
10. Roast the steak for 4 minutes on the medium heat.
11. Then discard the bay leaf and peppercorns and transfer the pork steak in the serving plates.

Nutrition: calories 465, fat 32.1, fiber 2, carbs 4, protein 38

Herbed Pork Belly

Prep time: 25 minutes
Cooking time: 24 hours
Servings: 8

Ingredients:

1-pound pork belly
1 teaspoon ground coriander
1 teaspoon ground ginger
1 tablespoon salt
1 teaspoon paprika
½ teaspoon chili flakes
1 teaspoon cilantro
1 tablespoon minced garlic

Directions:

1. Set Sous Vide water bath to 175 F and preheat it.
2. Rub the pork belly with the ground coriander, ground ginger, salt, paprika, chili flakes, cilantro, and minced garlic from the each side.
3. After this, put the pork belly in the plastic bag and seal the plastic bag.
4. Put the sealed plastic bag in the preheated water bath and cook it for 24 hours.
5. When the time is over – strain the liquid from the pork belly in the saucepan.
6. Put the pork belly on the wooden board.
7. Simmer the liquid from the pork belly until it is reduced in 2 times.
8. Then chill it gently and brush the pork belly.
9. Then slice the pork belly roughly.

Nutrition: calories 297, fat 30.2, fiber 0, carbs 1, protein 5

Wafu

Prep time: 25 minutes
Cooking time: 60 minutes
Servings: 2

Ingredients:

1 teaspoon garlic clove, sliced
12 oz pork steak
1 teaspoon salt
1 teaspoon ground white pepper
1 oz olive oil
1 tablespoon sunflower oil
2 oz daikon, grated
2 teaspoon ponzu

Directions:

1. Cut the pork steak into 2 parts and beat the pork steaks gently.
2. Then put the prepared meat in the plastic bag.
3. Add the salt, ground white pepper, and olive oil.
4. Close the plastic bag and seal it.
5. Preheat the water bath to 150 F.
6. Put the sealed plastic bag in the preheated water bath and cook it for 30 minutes.
7. Then remove the plastic bag from the water bath and open it – add the grated daikon and ponzu and close it again.
8. Continue to cook the pork steak for 30 minutes more.
9. The sprinkle the skillet with the sunflower oil and preheat it.
10. Transfer the content of the plastic bag in the preheated sunflower oil and roast the meat for 2 minutes on the each side on the medium heat.
11. Serve it!

Nutrition: calories 772, fat 59.3, fiber 0, carbs 7, protein 51

Red Wine Steak

Prep time: 20 minutes
Cooking time: 2 hours
Servings: 2

Ingredients:

1-pound pork steak
1 cup red wine
1 tablespoon salt
1 tablespoon ground black pepper
2 teaspoon butter
¼ teaspoon ground nutmeg
1 teaspoon sugar

Directions:

1. Combine the red wine with the salt, ground black pepper, ground nutmeg, and sugar.
2. Stir the liquid with the help of the spoon till sugar and salt are dissolved.
3. After this, put the pork steak in the plastic bag.
4. Add the red wine liquid and close the bag.
5. Vacuum the plastic bag and put it in the preheated to 131 F water bath.
6. Cook the pork steak for 2 hours.
7. When the time is over – strain the pork steak to get rid of the liquid.
8. Then toss the butter in the skillet and preheat it to the high heat.
9. Then reduce the heat to the medium level and put the pork steak there.
10. Cook it for 6 minutes total.
11. After this, cut the pork steak into 2 servings.

Nutrition: calories 678, fat 44.1, fiber 0, carbs 4, protein 57

Pork Steak in Duck Fat

Prep time: 15 minutes
Cooking time: 1.5 hour
Servings: 4

Ingredients:

15 oz pork steak
4 tablespoon duck fat
1 carrot
½ onion
1 tablespoon salt
¼ cup water
1 teaspoon ground red pepper
2 garlic cloves, peeled
1 thyme sprig

Directions:

1. Preheat Sous Vide water bath to 150 F.
2. Meanwhile, Pour water into the saucepan and preheat it well.
3. Then remove the preheated water from the heat and add the duck fat.
4. Then chop the carrot and onion roughly and add them to the water mixture.
5. Add the ground red pepper, peeled garlic cloves, and thyme sprig.
6. Stir the mixture till the duck fat is dissolved and pour it into the plastic bag.
7. Add the pork steak and close the plastic bag.
8. After this, seal the plastic bag and put it in the prepared water bath.
9. Cook the pork steak for 1.5 hours.
10. When the time is over – remove the plastic bag from the water bath and discard the pork steak from the duck fat mixture.

11. Transfer the pork steak in the serving plates and serve it with the cooked carrot and onion from the plastic bag.
12. Enjoy!

Nutrition: calories 858, fat 79.1, fiber 1, carbs 19, protein 19

Medium Rare Beef Steak

Prep time: 15 minutes
Cooking time: 2 hours
Servings: 5

Ingredients:

2-pound beef steak
½ teaspoon peppercorn
½ tablespoon salt
1 teaspoon oregano
1 teaspoon lemon zest
¼ teaspoon chili flakes
3 tablespoon olive oil
1 tablespoon butter

Directions:

1. Set Sous Vide water bath to 131 F and preheat it.
2. Meanwhile, separate the beef steak into 5 parts.
3. After this, sprinkle every steak part with the salt, oregano, lemon zest, and chili flakes,
4. Massage the meat gently with the help of the fingertips.
5. After this, take 2 plastic bags and put the beef steaks there.
6. Add peppercorn and olive oil. Close the plastic bags.
7. Then seal the plastic bags using the vacuum method.
8. Put the plastic bags in the preheated water bath and cook the meat for 2 hours.
9. When the time is over – discard the meat from the plastic bags.
10. Then toss the butter in the pan and melt it.
11. Put the beef steak in the preheated butter and cook them on the medium heat for 2 minutes from the both sides.
12. Serve the dish immediately.

13. Taste it!

Nutrition: calories 350, fat 20.7, fiber 0, carbs 0, protein 38

Desserts

Vanilla Chocolate Mousse

Prep time: 25 minutes
Cooking time: 1 hour
Servings: 3

Ingredients:

1 teaspoon vanilla extract
2 oz wine vinegar
1/3 cup chocolate chips
4 tablespoon caster sugar
1 tablespoon lemon zest
1 cup milk

Directions:

1. Set Sous Vide water bath to173 F.
2. Pour the milk in the plastic bag and add the wine vinegar.
3. Close the plastic bag and seal it.
4. Then transfer the sealed plastic bag in the preheated water bath and cook the mixture for 1 hour.
5. Meanwhile, put the chocolate chips in the bowl.
6. Make the water bath and put the bowl with the chocolate chips in the water bath.
7. Preheat the chocolate chips until they start to melt.
8. Then add the caster sugar and lemon zest. Mix it up.
9. Maintain the chocolate chips mixture warm.
10. When the time is over – remove the milk mixture from the water bath.
11. Strain the mixture to get rid of the excess liquid. Use the cheesecloth for this step.
12. After this, combine the milk mixture with the chocolate mixture and whisk it.
13. Put the cooked mousse in the ramekins and refrigerate them.
14. Enjoy!

Nutrition: calories 233, fat 8.8, fiber 1, carbs 33, protein 4

Melted Pineapple with Rum

Prep time: 15 minutes
Cooking time: 2 hours
Servings: 4

Ingredients:

1-pound pineapple
¼ teaspoon ground ginger
¼ teaspoon nutmeg
1 cup rum
2 teaspoon sugar

Directions:

1. Prepare the pineapple: peel it and chop into the medium cubes.
2. Then transfer the pineapple cubes in the plastic bag.
3. Sprinkle the pineapple with the ground ginger and nutmeg.
4. Add sugar and pour rum.
5. Close the plastic bag and seal it using the water immersion technique.
6. Preheat Sous Vide water bath to 136 F.
7. Put the sealed pineapple cubes in the preheated water bath and cook the dessert for 2 hours.
8. When the time is over – remove the plastic bag from the water bath.
9. Open the plastic bag and strain the liquid from it.
10. Put the cooked pineapple cubes in the big glass jar. Add the remaining rum liquid.
11. Close the jar lid and keep the dessert in the fridge.
12. Enjoy!

Nutrition: calories 203, fat 0.2, fiber 1, carbs 19, protein 1

Classic Crème Brule

Prep time: 20 minutes
Cooking time: 47 minutes
Servings: 5

Ingredients:

2 cup heavy cream
6 egg yolks
1 teaspoon vanilla sugar
4 tablespoon sugar
1 teaspoon vanilla extract

Directions:

1. Whisk the yolks with the vanilla sugar, sugar, and vanilla extract.
2. When you get the lemon color mixture – leave it.
3. Whip the heavy cream and then combine them with the egg yolk mixture.
4. Stir it carefully and pour the liquid into the saucepan.
5. Preheat the crème Brule mixture until it starts to boil. Stir the egg yolk mixture constantly.
6. Preheat Sous Vide water bath to 196 F.
7. When the crème Brule mixture is cooked – remove it from the heat.
8. Chill the crème Brule mixture using the ice bath.
9. When the crème Brule liquid is chilled – pour it into the mason jars.
10. Close the mason jars lids and put the vessels in the preheated water bath.
11. Cook the crème Brule for 47 minutes.
12. When the crème Brule is cooked – remove the mason jars from the water bath.
13. Chill the crème Brule gently.
14. Enjoy!

Nutrition: calories 258, fat 23.2, fiber 0, carbs 9, protein 4

Sweet Rice Pudding with Almond Milk

Prep time: 10 minutes
Cooking time: 3.5 hours
Servings: 4

Ingredients:

2 cup milk
1 cup almond milk
1 cup white rice
4 tablespoon sugar
1 teaspoon vanilla extract
1 tablespoon coconut
2 tablespoon cornstarch
1/3 teaspoon salt

Directions:

1. Set Sous Vide water bath to 181 F and preheat it.
2. Meanwhile, pour the milk and almond milk in the plastic bag.
3. Add the white rice and sugar.
4. After this, add the vanilla extract and coconut.
5. Add the cornstarch and shake the mixture gently.
6. Sprinkle the liquid mixture with the salt and close the plastic bag.
7. Seal the plastic bag using the water immersion technique.
8. Transfer the sealed plastic bag in the water bath and cook the rice pudding for 3.5 hours.
9. When the sweet rice pudding is cooked – transfer it to the serving bowls.
10. Serve the dish immediately and enjoy!

Nutrition: calories 310, fat 5, fiber 2, carbs 58, protein 7

Chocolate Cake

Prep time: 15 minutes
Cooking time: 3.5 hours
Servings: 6

Ingredients:

3 eggs
3 egg yolks
1 cup flour
1/3 cup cocoa powder
¼ teaspoon salt
¼ cup sugar
1 teaspoon vanilla extract
½ cup heavy cream
1 teaspoon lemon zest
1 tablespoon apple cider vinegar
½ teaspoon butter

Directions:

1. Beat the eggs in the mixer bowl.
2. Add the egg yolk and sugar.
3. Mix the mixture up until it is homogenous.
4. After this, add salt, cocoa powder, flour, vanilla extract, heavy cream, lemon zest, apple cider vinegar, and butter.
5. Mix the dough carefully until you get the smooth texture.
6. Then set Sous Vide water bath to 194 F and preheat it.
7. Transfer the chocolate dough mixture in the 6 mason jars and close them.
8. Put the mason jars in the preheated water bath and cook the chocolate cakes for 3.5 hours.
9. After this, remove the mason jars from the water bath and check if the cakes are cooked.
10. Then chill the dessert gently.

11. Enjoy!

Nutrition: calories 235, fat 11.9, fiber 2, carbs 24, protein 9

Chia Jar

Prep time: 10 minutes
Cooking time: 1.5 hours
Servings: 3

Ingredients:

2 tablespoon maple syrup
½ cup chia seeds
1 cup whole milk
½ teaspoon vanilla extract
¼ cup raspberries

Directions:

1. Combine the maple syrup, vanilla extract, and milk together in the big bowl.
2. Stir the mixture well to make it homogenous.
3. Then set Sous Vide water bath to 180 F.
4. Pour the whole milk mixture into the plastic bag.
5. Add the chia seeds and mix the mixture up.
6. Pour the chia mixture into the jars and close the lids.
7. Put the prepared mason jars in the preheated water bath.
8. Cook the chia jars for 1.5 hours.
9. When the time is over – discard the chia jars from the water bath.
10. Then open the lids and add the raspberries in every jar.
11. Serve the dish warm or keep it in the fridge, not more than 2 days!
12. Taste it!

Nutrition: calories 534, fat 28.2, fiber 29, carbs 60, protein 16

Honey Pears

Prep time: 15 minutes
Cooking time: 33 minutes
Servings: 4

Ingredients:

1-pound pear (4 pears)
3 tablespoon liquid honey
2 tablespoon butter
¼ cup cream
1/3 teaspoon nutmeg
1 tablespoon vanilla extract

Directions:

1. Cut the pears crosswise and remove the seeds from every half.
2. Set Sous Vide water bath to 174 F and preheat it.
3. After this, melt the butter and combine it with the liquid honey.
4. Add the cream, nutmeg, and vanilla extract.
5. Whisk the mixture using the hand whisker.
6. After this, put the pear halves in 2 plastic bags (2 pears per 1 bag).
7. Add the honey mixture to every plastic bag.
8. Close the plastic bags and seal them using the vacuum method.
9. Put the plastic bags in the water bath and cook the dessert for 33 minutes.
10. When the dish is cooked – transfer it to the big serving bowl.
11. Chill it for 1-2 minutes and serve.
12. Enjoy!

Nutrition: calories 186, fat 9, fiber 4, carbs 26, protein 1

Pumpkin Pie

Prep time: 25 minutes
Cooking time: 1.25 hour
Servings: 4

Ingredients:

7 oz graham crackers
5 tablespoon butter
¼ cup sugar
7 oz pumpkin, canned
¼ teaspoon salt
½ cup heavy cream
1 teaspoon ground cinnamon
1 teaspoon ground ginger
½ teaspoon ground nutmeg
2 tablespoon almond flour

Directions:

1. Put the canned pumpkin in the mixer bowl.
2. Add the salt, sugar, heavy cream, ground cinnamon, ground ginger, and ground nutmeg.
3. After this, add the almond flour and mix it up until the mixture is smooth.
4. Set Sous Vide water bath to 177 F and preheat it.
5. Pour the pumpkin mixture into the plastic bag.
6. Close the plastic bag and seal it.
7. After this, put the pumpkin mixture in the preheated water bath and cook it for 1.25 hour.
8. Meanwhile, crush the graham crackers and combine them with butter.
9. Mix the mixture to get the crust dough.
10. Then take the cake mold and make the pie crust there.
11. Put the cake mold with the pie crust in the freezer.
12. After this, preheat the oven to 360 F.

13. When the pumpkin mixture is cooked – remove it from the water bath and chill gently.
14. Then remove the pie crust from the freezer.
15. Pour the pumpkin mixture into the pie crust.
16. Then put the pie in the preheated oven.
17. Cook the dish for 10 minutes.
18. When the time is over – remove the pie from the oven and chill it for at least 10 minutes.
19. Slice the pumpkin pie.
20. Serve it!

Nutrition: calories 646, fat 35.3, fiber 11, carbs 73, protein 13

Strawberry Cheesecake

Prep time: 18 minutes
Cooking time: 1 hour 15 minutes
Servings: 4

Ingredients:

½ cup cottage cheese
½ cup cream cheese
½ cup sugar
4 eggs
3 tablespoon strawberry jam
2 tablespoon milk
1 tablespoon flour
1 teaspoon orange zest

Directions:

1. Combine the cream cheese and cottage cheese together in the big bowl.
2. Mix the mixture with the help of the hand mixer until it is smooth and homogenous.
3. Then add sugar and beat the eggs.
4. Mix the mixture well for 3 minutes on the maximum speed.
5. Then add the strawberry jam and milk.
6. Sprinkle the cheese mixture with the flour and orange zest.
7. Mix it up for 1 minute more. The prepared mixture should have smooth but soft texture.
8. Preheat the water bath to 180 F.
9. Transfer the cheesecake mixture into the mason jars. Close the lids.
10. Put the cheesecakes in the preheated water bath.
11. Cook the dessert for 1 hour and 15 minutes.
12. After this, chill the mason jars with the cheesecake and put them in the fridge for 10 minutes.

13. Serve and enjoy!

Nutrition: calories 308, fat 19.6, fiber 0, carbs 18, protein 15

Walnut Pie

Prep time: 20 minutes
Cooking time: 3 hours
Servings: 8

Ingredients:

½ cup walnuts, crushed
1 cup flour
½ cup heavy cream
½ teaspoon baking soda
1 tablespoon apple cider vinegar
¼ teaspoon salt
4 tablespoon caster sugar
1 egg
2 teaspoon butter

Directions:

1. Beat the egg in the bowl and whisk it using the hand whisker.
2. After this, add the heavy cream and caster sugar.
3. Keep whisking the mixture till it is homogenous.
4. Then add the baking soda and apple cider vinegar.
5. Sprinkle the liquid mixture with the butter and salt. Add the flour and crushed walnuts.
6. Knead the homogeneous but little bit liquid dough.
7. Preheat Sous Vide water bath to 175 F.
8. Pour the walnut pie dough into the glass jars and close them with the lids.
9. Then put the jars in the preheated water bath.
10. Cook the walnut pie for 3 hours.
11. When the walnut pie is cooked – remove it from the water bath.
12. Serve the cooked dessert in the glass jars. Eat the pie using the teaspoon.
13. Enjoy!

Nutrition: calories 157, fat 8.4, fiber 1, carbs 17, protein 4

Apple Cobbler

Prep time: 21 minutes
Cooking time: 3.5 hours
Servings: 5

Ingredients:

2 green apples
1 cup milk
7 tablespoon flour
4 tablespoon brown sugar
1 teaspoon vanilla extract
1 teaspoon butter
1 teaspoon ground cardamom

Directions:

1. Peel the apples and cut them into the cubes.
2. Then combine the apple cubes with the brown sugar and milk.
3. Add vanilla extract and ground cardamom. Stir it gently with the help of the spoon.
4. Add the flour and butter.
5. Mix it up until the mixture is homogenous. You can combine the milk with the flour separately to make the texture softer and after this, combine it with the apples.
6. Then preheat water bath to 191 F.
7. Pour the apple cobbler mixture in 5 mason jars. Close the lids.
8. Put the apple cobbler jars in the water bath.
9. Cook the dish for 3.5 hours.
10. When the time is over – chill the apple cobbler – use the ice bath for this step.
11. Serve the dish and enjoy!

Nutrition: calories 201, fat 2.6, fiber 2, carbs 43, protein 3

Milk Kheer

Prep time: 25 minutes
Cooking time: 3 hours
Servings: 4

Ingredients:

¼ cup rice
2 tablespoon sugar
¼ cup milk
1 teaspoon vanilla extract
¼ cup coconut milk
3 tablespoon almond, crushed
4 cardamom pods

Directions:

1. Set Sous Vide water bath to 181 F.
2. Take the mason jars and put the rice in every of them.
3. After this, take the big bowl and combine the milk, vanilla extract, sugar, coconut milk, and mix the liquid till the sugar is dissolved.
4. After this, pour the milk mixture into the rice jars.
5. Then sprinkle every rice jar with the crushed almond and add the cardamom pods.
6. Close the glass jar lids.
7. After this, transfer the glass jars in the preheated water bath and cook the milk kheer for 3 hours.
8. Meanwhile, prepare the ice bath: put the ice cubes in the bowl.
9. When the milk kheer is cooked – transfer the glass jars in the prepared ice bath and chill it well.
10. After this, open the glass jars and mix the dish well with the help of the spoon.

Nutrition: calories 91, fat 6.1, fiber 2, carbs 10, protein 2

Chocolate Cupcakes

Prep time: 20 minutes
Cooking time: 3 hours
Servings: 6

Ingredients:

3 tablespoon cocoa powder
1 teaspoon baking soda
1 teaspoon apple cider vinegar
1/3 teaspoon salt
4 tablespoon sugar
½ cup heavy cream
1 egg
5 tablespoon butter
1 cup flour
1 teaspoon vanilla extract

Directions:

1. Combine the cocoa powder, baking soda, salt, sugar, and flour in the bowl.
2. Stir the dried mixture gently with the help of the fork.
3. After this, take the separated bowl and pour the heavy cream there.
4. Beat the egg in the heavy cream and add butter.
5. Then sprinkle the mixture with the vanilla extract and whisk the mass until it is homogenous.
6. After this, combine the dry mixture and liquid mixture together.
7. Add the apple cider vinegar and stir it till you get the smooth texture of the dough.
8. Set Sous Vide water bath t 194 F.
9. Put the dough in 6 mason jars and close the lids.
10. After this, put the mason jars with the chocolate dough in the preheated water bath and cook them for 3 hours.

11. When the time is over – serve the cupcakes immediately or sprinkle them with the icing.
12. Enjoy!

Nutrition: calories 211, fat 11.8, fiber 1, carbs 23, protein 4

Sous Vide Flan

Prep time: 25 minutes
Cooking time: 2 hours
Servings: 5

Ingredients:

11 oz condensed milk
5 eggs
6 oz coconut milk
6 oz sugar
4 oz water
6 tablespoon coconut flakes

Directions:

1. Preheat Sous Vide water bath to 181 F.
2. Meanwhile, combine the condensed milk and coconut milk together.
3. Beat the eggs into the mixture and mix it until you get the homogeneous liquid texture of the mass.
4. Then preheat the skillet well and put the sugar there.
5. Melt the sugar and add water. Stir it carefully to get the sticky caramel.
6. After this, pour cooked caramel in every glass jar.
7. Then add the condensed milk mixture and close the lids.
8. Put the jars in the preheated water bath and cook the flan for 2 hours.
9. Meanwhile, preheat the oven to 365 F.
10. Sprinkle the tray with the coconut flakes and bake them in the preheated oven for 2 minutes. Stir them frequently.
11. Then chill the coconut flakes.
12. When the flan is cooked – remove the jars from the water bath and chill little.
13. Put the flan jars in the fridge and chill overnight.

14. Then sprinkle the cooked flan with the baked coconut flakes.
15. Enjoy!

Nutrition: calories 407, fat 21.6, fiber 1, carbs 43, protein 12

Berry Mousse

Prep time: 15 minutes
Cooking time: 1 hour
Servings: 6

Ingredients:

1 cup cream cheese
½ cup strawberry
½ cup raspberry
½ cup sugar
1 cup milk
1 tablespoon flour
2 tablespoon cornstarch
¼ teaspoon salt
1 teaspoon ground ginger
1 tablespoon cocoa powder

Directions:

1. Put the strawberries and raspberries in the blender.
2. Add sugar, salt, and ground ginger.
3. Blend the mixture well till you get the smooth texture.
4. After this, add the cream cheese, milk, flour, cornstarch, and cocoa powder and blend it well.
5. When the uncooked mousse mixture is cooked – pour it into the 6 glass jars and close with the lids.
6. Set Sous Vide water bath to 172 F.
7. When the water bath is preheated – put the glass jars with the mousse there.
8. Cook the dish for 1 hour.
9. After this, chill the berry mousse carefully.
10. Enjoy!

Nutrition: calories 216, fat 13, fiber 1, carbs 22, protein 5

Berry Compote

Prep time: 15 minutes
Cooking time: 1 hour
Servings: 6

Ingredients:

½ cup lemon juice
1 cup blackberries
1 cup sugar
1 tablespoon fresh mint
1 cup orange juice
1 tablespoon cornstarch

Directions:

1. Smash the blackberries with the help of the fork well.
2. After this, add the sugar and cornstarch.
3. Mix the mixture up and add the orange juice.
4. Stir the berry mixture and pour it in the plastic bag.
5. Add the fresh mint.
6. Seal the plastic bag using the vacuum method.
7. Preheat Sous Vide water bath to 175 F.
8. Put the sealed plastic bag with the compote in the preheated water bath and cook it for 1 hour.
9. When the time is over – transfer the berry compote in the big glass jar.
10. Discard the fresh mint and serve the dessert.
11. Enjoy!

Nutrition: calories 164, fat 1, fiber 2, carbs 39, protein 1

Green Gelato

Prep time: 25 minutes
Cooking time: 1 hour
Servings: 4

Ingredients:

2 tablespoon fresh mint
1 teaspoon vanilla extract
7 egg yolks
½ cup milk
1 cup heavy cream
4 tablespoon pistachio, crushed
¼ teaspoon nutmeg

Directions:

1. Put the fresh mint in the blender and blend it until it is smooth.
2. Then add the egg yolks and vanilla extract.
3. Keep mixing the mixture for 1 minute on the high speed.
4. After this, add the milk and heavy cream.
5. Then add the crushed pistachios and nutmeg.
6. Mix the mixture until it is homogenous.
7. Preheat the water bath to 179 F.
8. Pour the prepared gelato mixture in the saucepan.
9. Put the saucepan on the medium heat and cook it for 4 minutes.
10. Stir it constantly.
11. After this, transfer the gelato mixture in the plastic bag.
12. Seal the plastic bag and transfer it in the preheated water bath.
13. Cook the gelato for 1 hour.
14. When the time is over – transfer the gelato to the bowl and stir it.
15. Chill the gelato using the ice bath.

16. Enjoy!

Nutrition: calories 356, fat 26.1, fiber 1, carbs 22, protein 8

Vanilla Mini Cake

Prep time: 30 minutes
Cooking time: 3 hours
Servings: 6

Ingredients:

1 cup sugar
1 cup flour
6 eggs
1 teaspoon vanilla extract
1 teaspoon ground cinnamon
2 tablespoon butter

Directions:

1. Crack the eggs into the bowl and whisk them with the help of the hand whisker.
2. Add the sugar, flour, vanilla extract, ground cinnamon, and butter.
3. Mix the mixture with the help of the hand mixer for 5 minutes on the medium speed.
4. After this, leave the vanilla dough for 10 minutes.
5. Meanwhile, preheat the water bath to 195 F.
6. Pour the vanilla cake dough into 6 mason jars.
7. Close the mason jar lids and transfer the cakes in the preheated water bath.
8. Cook the cakes for 3 hours.
9. When the time is over remove the mini cakes from the water bath and leave them for 10 minutes to chill.
10. After this, remove the mini cakes from the mason jars and serve the dessert.
11. Enjoy!

Nutrition: calories 307, fat 13.7, fiber 1, carbs 34, protein 11

Conclusion

Thanks for making it through to the end of this book, let's hope it was informative and able to provide you with all of the tools you need to achieve your goals whatever they may be.

The next step is to start trying out the sous vide cooking method for yourself. This method of cooking is simple to work with, and you really only need a few supplies to get it all started. Once everything is in order, you will be able to make some of the best meals of your life, without having to worry about the meal overcooking or something else going wrong like you do with some of your other cooking methods.

This book is going to take some time to discuss the sous vide cooking method and how you can make it your own. Sous vide may sound complicated, but it is actually a pretty easy cooking method that just requires a hot water bath that maintains the same temperature throughout the whole cooking process. It has been really popular in restaurants for many years. When you are done reading through this book, you are sure to find that sous vide cooking is a great option.

When you are ready to get started with sous vide cooking in your own home and learning how to create restaurant style meals without all the headache, make sure to check out this book to learn how to get started.

Bon Appetit!

One Last Thing... Did You Enjoy the Book?

If so, then let me know by leaving a review on Amazon! Reviews are the lifeblood of independent authors. I would appreciate even a few words from you!

If you did not like the book, then please tell me! Email me at lizard.publishing@gmail.com and let me know what you didn't like. Perhaps I can change it. In today's world, a book doesn't have to be stagnant. It should be improved with time and feedback from readers like you. You can impact this book, and I welcome your feedback. Help me make this book better for everyone!

Printed in Great Britain
by Amazon